ACCIDENT AND EMERGENCY
Diagnosis and Management

Accident and Emergency Diagnosis and Management

Third edition

ANTHONY F.T. BROWN
MBChB, FRCP, FRICS(Ed), FACEM, FFAEM

*Staff Specialist, Department of Emergency Medicine, Royal Brisbane Hospital
Clinical Associate Professor, Faculty of Medicine, University of Queensland, Brisbane, Queensland, Australia*

(Formerly: Accident and Emergency Department, Addenbrooke's Hospital, Cambridge, England)

Foreword to the first edition
Dr H. Baderman FRCP
Consultant, Accident and Emergency Department, University College Hospital, London

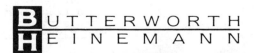

Butterworth-Heinemann
Linacre House, Jordan Hill, Oxford OX2 8DP
225 Wildwood Avenue, Woburn, MA 01801-2041
A division of Reed Educational and Professional Publishing Ltd

$\mathcal{R}$ A member of the Reed Elsevier plc group

OXFORD   BOSTON   JOHANNESBURG
MELBOURNE   NEW DELHI   SINGAPORE

First published 1987
Reprinted 1988, 1990 (twice)
Second edition 1992
Reprinted 1992, 1993 (twice), 1994, 1995 (twice), 1996
Third edition 1996
Reprinted 1998 (twice)

British Library Cataloguing in Publication Data
Brown, Anthony F. T.
  Accident and emergancy: diagnosis and management - 3rd ed.
  1. Emergency medicine
  I. Title
  616'.025
ISBN 0 7506 2233 4

Library of Congress Cataloguing in Publication Data
Brown, Anthony F. T.
  Accident adn emergency: diagnosis and management?Anthony F. T.
  Brown. - 3rd ed.
  p. cm.
  Includes bibliographical references and index.
  ISBN 0 7506 2233 4
  1. Emergency medicine - Handbooks, manuals, etc. I. Title
  [DNLM: 1. Emergencies - handbooks. WB 39 B877a 1996]
  RC86.8.B76   96-3796
  616.02'5--dc20   CIP

Composition by Scribe Design, Gillingham, Kent
Printed and bound in Great Britain

PLANT A TREE

FOR EVERY TITLE THAT WE PUBLISH, BUTTERWORTH-HEINEMANN
WILL PAY FOR BTCV TO PLANT AND CARE FOR A TREE.

100156124I

Contents

SECTION V ENT emergencies

SECTION VI Ophthalmic emergencies

Foreword to the first edition

The specialty of accident and emergency medicine has long since come of age. The A & E department is recognized now as providing a crucial service, sitting as it does at the interface between the community and the hospital and seeing literally a multitude of patients with conditions that arise in every specialty in medicine and some that defy classification, far less resolution. The aim, of course, is to provide a high standard of care, speedily and with sensitivity and kindness to all these patients, minor or major cases, the elderly and the very young, clear-headed or confused, meek or aggressive. The unexpected and the unsuspected is always likely to be the next patient. And the risk of making a mistake in diagnosis or management is ever-present. All-in-all, a tall order for the doctors working in these departments, a huge majority of whom are within a year or two of qualification.

A good handbook of differential diagnosis and initial management is as essential a piece of our everyday equipment as a stethoscope or x-ray viewing box and should be used at least as frequently as either. Anthony Brown writes from experience and commitment. His new manual fits into the pocket of our white coats but should be taken out and consulted frequently for our instruction, and our patients' benefit.

Howard Baderman FRCP
Consultant
A & E Department
University College Hospital
London

Dedication

To Mum and Dad with love

Preface to the third edition

This new edition is again primarily written for senior house officers in the A & E department. It aims to provide didactic, practical advice in an easily read format on the important points in the history, examination, investigation and immediate management of every patient — however unusual, complex or unexpected the presentation.

In addition, senior A & E staff, general practitioners, nurses and medical students working in A & E departments will also benefit from the same advice by creating teamwork from this shared knowledge, as the basis for quality emergency care.

The entire text has been updated with many parts rewritten. Completely new topics include adenosine, acid–base disturbances, domestic violence, hyperosmolar nonketotic coma, intraosseous infusion and knee aspiration to name but a few. The latest UK tetanus prophylaxis guidelines, European Resuscitation Council CPR guidelines and the revised CDC classification system for human immunodeficiency virus infection reflect the need to remain in the forefront of developments in acute care.

Whatever the outcome of the issues presently besetting the specialty of A & E medicine, such as manpower and rosters, the rationalisation of resources and the interface with primary care, a helpful, familiar core A & E handbook will remain essential. It is with this in mind that I offer a new edition to my colleagues.

Anthony F.T. Brown
October 1995

Preface to the first edition

This book is primarily written for the junior doctor new to the A & E department, and is designed to fit the white coat pocket, to be available at all times. It will also assist general practitioners in the assessment of most acute problems seen in practice and perhaps help to bridge the interface between hospital and community care. This book should also appeal to medical students seeking a succinct guide to acute patient care. Finally, I hope it will also help nurses, ambulance personnel and other health workers involved in the various branches of emergency care.

I have written throughout in the same format. First 'diagnosis', emphasising the salient features in the history and examination and indicating which bedside or laboratory tests are required. This is followed by 'management' which describes essential immediate care first (and details on how to carry out any practical procedures), and then further treatment including precise details of drug dosages and common sources of error.

I have indicated when senior help is required; which patients to refer immediately, which to send home and which need outpatient follow-up. It is so often deciding who to send home, rather than who to refer, that worries the doctor new to A & E work!

I appreciate that there is no substitute for experience, but much initial indecision can be due to a lack of an orderly approach to the plethora of conditions seen daily in a busy department. I therefore offer a framework on which to build expertise. Further knowledge will be gained from regular teaching, audit, research and journal meetings held in the department and by listening to the advice of the senior staff.

The rich variety of work in modern A & E departments reflects the growing popularity of the specialty. Two factors in the success and enjoyment a new doctor gains from his work are confidence and a warm, humane approach. Whilst the latter cannot simply be taught, the former may assuredly be developed from well-structured knowledge. It is to this end that I offer this small volume to my colleagues.

Anthony F. T. Brown
February 1987

Acknowledgements

I would like to recognise in particular the following A & E specialists who made so many useful comments and helpful suggestions for this new edition: Mr John Heyworth, Dr Mike Beckett and Dr Geoff Hughes. Also, Mr Peter London for his pre-eminent contribution with such clarity of thought. I bow to their knowledge and expertise so readily shared. Thank you. In addition, thanks to Dr Ralph Hanson in Sydney for his help with the paediatrics section.

Thanks also to Sheila Sellars and Catherine Zank-McKelvey at Butterworth-Heinemann for their advice and encouragement.

Finally, I am indebted to Judy Shanks who typed the entire text, and whose accuracy, reliability and capacity to meet increasingly impossible deadlines established the basis for the successful completion of the many drafts of this new work.

Anthony F.T. Brown
October 1995

MEDICAL EMERGENCIES

CARDIOPULMONARY RESUSCITATION

DIAGNOSIS

The only essential feature in making a diagnosis of cardiac arrest is the absence of a pulse in a large artery such as the carotid or the femoral, although the following may be present:

(1) a brief tonic grand mal fit or unresponsiveness;
(2) gasping or absent breathing;
(3) pallor or cyanosis;
(4) dilated pupils.

MANAGEMENT

This is based on the European Resuscitation Council Guidelines 1992.[1,2]

(1) (i)   The first person on the scene stays with the patient and commences resuscitation, making a note of the time.

    (ii) The second person summons help and organises the arrival of equipment, then assists with the resuscitation.

(2) *Immediate actions.* The aim is to maintain oxygenation of the brain and heart until a stable cardiac output is achieved.

    (i)   Lay the patient flat on a hard surface such as a trolley. If the patient is on the floor and enough people are available, lift the patient on to a trolley to facilitate the resuscitation procedure.

    (ii) Give one sharp thump to the precordium in witnessed or monitored arrests.

    (iii) Open the airway by tilting the head and lifting the chin to prevent the tongue from occluding the larynx.

    (iv) Remove any obvious obstruction including loose dentures from the mouth, but leave well-fitting dentures in place.

    (v) Commence assisted ventilation.

      (vi)   Commence external cardiac massage.

(3) *Assisted ventilation.*
- (i) Start mouth-to-mouth or mouth-to-mask respiration, using a Laerdal Pocket Mask.
- (ii) An Ambu or Laerdal bag with oxygen reservoir attached and face mask may be used by a trained person after first inserting an oropharyngeal (Guedel) airway.
- (iii) If the chest fails to inflate, check for leaks around the mask or airway then consider obstruction of the upper airway (see page 30).

Note: adequate oxygenation is achieved by the above measures. Attempts at endotracheal intubation should only be made by doctors experienced in the technique.

(4) *External cardiac massage.*
- (i) Place the heel of the hand over the middle of the lower half of the sternum. Place the other hand on top, keeping the arms straight and using a rocking movement.
- (ii) Depress the sternum 4–5 cm at a rate of about 80 compressions per minute.
- (iii) It is unnecessary to synchronise massage with ventilation if there are two operators. If still alone, perform 15 compressions to every 2 ventilations. This should create a palpable femoral pulse.
- (iv) In small children, one hand only should be used at a rate of 100 compressions per minute; in infants, the tips of two fingers also at a rate of 100 compressions per minute.

Note: avoid using excessive force causing rib fractures, flail chest, liver lacerations, etc.

(5) *Definitive treatment.*
- (i) After confirming the diagnosis of cardiac arrest, give the patient an immediate 200 J shock.
- (ii) Defibrillation:
  - (a) This is an emergency situation. Do not await ECG confirmation at this crucial stage in re-establishing the circulation.

(b) Remove all glyceryl trinitrate patches or ointment from the chest wall to prevent an explosion.

(c) Place one paddle below the outer half of the right clavicle, and the other just outside the usual position of the cardiac apex (V4–5 of the ECG).

(d) Ensure good contact is made using electrode jelly or a pad (never KY jelly) and firm pressure.

(e) Make sure that no one is touching the patient or bed. Give a warning when the shock is about to be delivered.

(6) Connect the ECG monitor and observe one of four possible traces:

(i)   Ventricular fibrillation or ventricular tachycardia (see page 5).

(ii) Asystole (see page 8).

(iii) Electromechanical dissociation (see page 8).

(7) Establish an initial intravenous line in the antecubital fossa and commence a normal saline infusion giving at least 20 ml to flush any drugs administered towards the heart.

(8) Unless the cardiac resuscitation is rapidly successful, establish a second intravenous line:

(i)   Ideally the line should be inserted into a central vein, either the external or internal jugular or the subclavian.

(ii) This central line should only be inserted by an anaesthetist or similarly skilled doctor, as inadvertent arterial puncture, haemothorax and pneumothorax may invalidate further resuscitation attempts.

(iii) Also, the central venous route poses additional serious hazards should thrombolytic therapy be indicated.

(iv) All drugs are then given via this central line.

(9) *Endotracheal intubation.* An anaesthetist or similarly skilled doctor should now insert a cuffed endotracheal tube. This improves oxygenation and prevents inhalation of vomit or blood from the mouth or stomach.

(i) Use an 8.5–9.5 mm diameter endotracheal tube in the adult male or a 7.5–8.5 mm diameter in the adult female.

(ii) Pass the tube between the vocal cords under direct vision, using a curved blade laryngoscope.

(iii) Inflate the cuff, connect the oxygen supply and check the correct position of the tube by auscultation, or end tidal carbon dioxide measurement. Tie the tube in place.

(10) Subsequent management depends on the cardiac rhythm and the patient's condition. Keep the ECG monitor attached to the patient at all times.

(11) *Ventricular fibrillation* (VF). Disorganised electrical activity that may be coarse (large amplitude) or fine (low amplitude). See Table 1 for a rapid overview of treatment.

    (i) Treat with immediate DC shocks:

        (a) Start at 200 J (2 J/kg in small children);

        (b) If no effect, repeat 200 J;

        (c) If no effect, give further DC shock at 360 J.

    (ii) If VF recurs, give 10 ml of 1 in 10 000 adrenaline (1 mg) i.v., 10 sequences of five compressions to one breath and repeat a set of three DC shocks at 360 J.

    (iii) If VF persists, repeat the above loop of adrenaline 1 mg, 10 compression/ventilation sequences and three DC shocks.

    (iv) If VF still persists repeat the loop a third time.

    (v) If VF still persists, consider an alkalising agent and one of the antiarrhythmic drugs:

        (a) *8.4% sodium bicarbonate.* Give up to 50 mmol (50 ml) i.v.

        (b) *Lignocaine.* Give a bolus of 1.5 mg/kg i.v., repeated up to a total of 3 mg/kg.

        (c) *Bretylium.* Give a bolus of 5 mg/kg i.v. Vials contain 50 mg/ml so give approximately 7 ml or 350 mg for a 70-kg patient. Repeat the DC shock. A second dose of 10 mg/kg may be given, repeated to a total of 30–35 mg/kg.

        (d) *Amiodarone.* Give a bolus of 5 mg/kg i.v. in 10–20 ml of 5% dextrose.

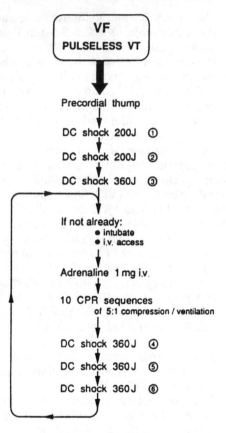

Notes: (i)   The interval between shocks 3 and 4 should not be >2 min.

          (ii) Adrenaline given during loop approx every 2–3 min.

          (iii) Continue loops for as long as defibrillation is indicated.

          (iv) After 3 loops consider:

                    ● an alkalising agent

                    ● an antiarrhythmic agent.

Table 1. Algorithm for ventricular fibrillation (VF) or pulseless ventricular tachycardia (VT). (Reproduced by kind permission of *Resuscitation*.)

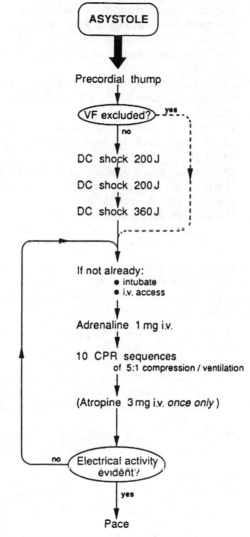

Table 2. Algorithm for asystole. (Reproduced by kind permission of *Resuscitation*.)

(vi)   Repeat three loops of adrenaline 1 mg, 10 compression/ventilation sequences and three DC shocks after each drug bolus. Try different paddle positions, even a change of defibrillator in refractory VF.

(12) *Asystole*. No electrical activity — check an ECG lead has not come off. See Table 2 for a rapid overview of treatment.

(i)   If ventricular fibrillation cannot be excluded, give up to three DC shocks immediately (see under 11 (i) above).

(ii)   Otherwise give 10 ml of 1 in 10 000 adrenaline (1 mg) i.v. followed by 10 sequences of five compressions to one breath.

(iii)   If no effect, give atropine 3 mg i.v. once only. This may relieve any vagal inhibition from intubation etc., that will have been augmented by hypoxia.

Note: if venous access is difficult (e.g. in small children), give atropine, adrenaline and lignocaine via the endotracheal tube at two to three times the intravenous dosage, diluted with normal saline to a total of 10 ml.

(iv)   If still in asystole the prognosis is very poor. However, if P waves or any other electrical activity are present, consider pacing:

(a)   A temporary transvenous pacemaker wire may be inserted blind via a central vein but ideally should be passed under x-ray guidance.

(b)   Or use an external (transcutaneous) pacemaker to maintain the cardiac output until a transvenous wire is inserted.

(v)   Otherwise, repeat the loop of adrenaline 1 mg and 10 compression/ventilation sequences.

(vi)   If still in asystole after three loops, give high-dose adrenaline 5 mg i.v.

(13) *Electromechanical dissociation*. Apparently coordinated waveform on the ECG but with no detectable cardiac output. Always consider causes requiring urgent treatment first, including tension pneumothorax, cardiac

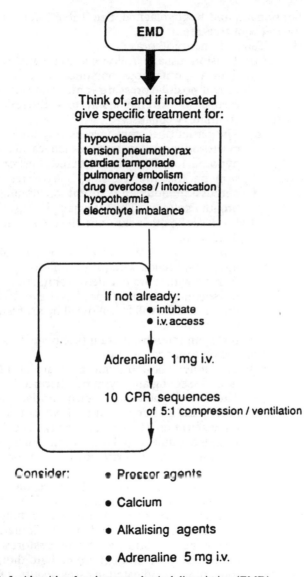

EMD

Think of, and if indicated
give specific treatment for:

hypovolaemia
tension pneumothorax
cardiac tamponade
pulmonary embolism
drug overdose / intoxication
hyopothermia
electrolyte imbalance

If not already:
- intubate
- i.v. access

Adrenaline 1 mg i.v.

10 CPR sequences
of 5:1 compression / ventilation

Consider:
- Proccor agents
- Calcium
- Alkalising agents
- Adrenaline 5 mg i.v.

Table 3. Algorithm for electromechanical dissociation (EMD).
(Reproduced by kind permission of *Resuscitation*.)

tamponade and hypovolaemia. See Table 3 for a rapid overview of treatment.

(i) Tension pneumothorax:

   (a) Tension usually follows a traumatic rather than a spontaneous pneumothorax, particularly if positive pressure ventilation is used. It results in extreme respiratory distress and circulatory collapse.

   (b) The patient becomes increasingly breathless, cyanosed and develops a tachycardia with hypotension. There is decreased chest expansion on the affected side, a hyperresonant percussion note and absent or diminished breath sounds. The trachea is displaced towards the other side, and the neck veins are distended.

   (c) This is a life-threatening situation requiring immediate relief, without waiting for a CXR.

   (d) Insert a wide-bore needle or cannula through the second intercostal space in the midclavicular line. This will be followed by a whistle of air outwards.

   (e) Insert an intercostal drain (see page 24).

(ii) Cardiac tamponade:

   (a) This may follow trauma, myocardial infarction, dissecting aneurysm or pericarditis.

   (b) There is hypotension, tachycardia, pulsus paradoxus and engorged neck veins that rise on inspiration (Kussmaul's sign). The heart sounds are quiet and the apex beat impalpable.

   (c) If the patient is in *extremis*, perform pericardiocentesis:

   Insert a cardiac needle between the angle of the xiphisternum and the left costal margin, at 45° to the horizontal, aiming for the left shoulder (see Fig. 1). Sometimes aspirating as little as 50 ml restores the cardiac output, although immediate thoracotomy may be indicated in cases resulting from trauma (see page 156).

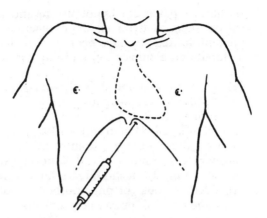

Fig. 1. Pericardial aspiration.

(iii) Hypovolaemia.
  (a) Severe blood loss following trauma, gastrointestinal haemorrhage, ruptured aortic aneurysm or ruptured ectopic pregnancy may cause cardiovascular collapse and cardiac arrest.
  (b) This must always be considered in cases of unexplained cardiovascular collapse.
  (c) Give fluid replacement rapidly and search for the source of bleeding. Call the surgical team urgently.
(iv) In the absence of the above causes of electromechanical dissociation:
  (a) Give 10 ml of 1 in 10 000 adrenaline (1 mg) i.v. followed by 10 sequences of five compressions to one breath.
  (b) Only use 10% calcium chloride 10 ml i.v. for hyperkalaemia, hypocalcaemia and overdose with calcium antagonist drugs.
(14) *Subsequent action*: it is important to continue effective external cardiac massage until the heartbeat is strong enough to produce a peripheral pulse.

(i) If there is persistent hypotension, and treatable causes such as hypoxia, hypovolaemia, tension pneumothorax, etc. have been excluded, consider a dobutamine infusion preferably via a central line:

    (a) Add dobutamine 250 mg to 500 ml of 5% dextrose, i.e. 500 µg/ml.

    (b) Infuse at 2–10 µg/kg per min or 0.3–1.4 ml/min (18–84 ml/h) for a 70-kg patient.

(ii) Transfer the patient to the intensive care unit or coronary care unit. The following investigations will be required, but should not delay transfer:

    (a) CXR to look for pneumothorax, pulmonary oedema and pulmonary collapse. Confirm correct positioning of the endotracheal tube and central line;

    (b) Blood gases;

    (c) Serum potassium and glucose;

    (d) 12-lead ECG.

(iii) The patient must be transferred with a trained nurse and preferably a doctor in attendance. A portable cardiac monitor, defibrillator, oxygen and suction should be available on the trolley.

(15) *When to stop*. The decision to cease further attempts at resuscitation is difficult and should only be made by the senior member of the cardiac arrest team.

Survival from cardiac arrest is greatest when:

(i) The event is witnessed.

(ii) A bystander starts resuscitation.

(iii) The heart arrests in ventricular fibrillation.

(iv) Defibrillation is carried out at an early stage.

Note: special consideration must be given to near drowning, hypothermia and acute poisoning (especially with tricyclic antidepressants). Full recovery has followed in apparently hopeless cases (fixed dilated pupils, asystole) with resuscitation prolonged for many hours.

CHEST PAIN

DIFFERENTIAL DIAGNOSIS

Consider the life-threatening diagnoses first:
(i)   myocardial infarction;
(ii)   pulmonary embolus;
(iii)   aortic dissection.
These three can present with a normal CXR and ECG and may therefore need to be referred on clinical suspicion alone. Always establish venous access, give 35% oxygen and attach a cardiac monitor and pulse oximeter to the patient. Other causes to consider include:
(iv)   pericarditis;
(v)   pleurisy;
(vi)   pneumonia;
(vii)   pneumothorax;
(viii) abdominal — oesophagitis, oesophageal rupture, gallbladder disease, etc;
(ix)   musculoskeletal and chest wall pain.

MYOCARDIAL INFARCTION (MI)

DIAGNOSIS

(1) Predisposing factors include cigarette smoking, hypertension, diabetes, hypercholesterolaemia and a positive family history.
(2) There may be a prior history of angina, myocardial infarction or heart failure.
(3) Typically the pain is central, crushing, retrosternal, usually lasting for 30 minutes or longer, unrelieved by sublingual nitrates and associated with anxiety, dyspnoea, nausea and vomiting.
(4) The pain radiates to the neck, jaw, one or both arms, the back and occasionally to the epigastrium, or may present at these sites alone.
(5) The patient may be clammy, sweaty, breathless and pale.

(6) The patient may present atypically with the complications of heart failure, cardiac arrhythmia, hypotension, systemic embolism or collapse. Alternatively, the patient may look deceptively well.

(7) Investigations that subsequently establish the underlying diagnosis include:

(i) ECG. Acute changes include convex ST elevation (acute injury), T-wave inversion (ischaemia) and the formation of Q waves (infarction).

    (a) Inferior MI causes changes in leads II, III and aVF.

    (b) Anterior MI causes changes in I, aVL and V1–V3 (anteroseptal) or V4–V6 (anterolateral).

    (c) True posterior MI causes mirror-image changes of tall R waves and ST depression in leads V1–V4.

(ii) Chest x-ray to exclude pulmonary oedema, cardiomegaly and atelectasis. Request a portable x-ray in the A & E department, providing this does not delay admission to the ward.

(iii) Raised cardiac enzymes such as creatine phosphokinase and MB isoenzymes.

MANAGEMENT

(1) Establish venous access with a heparinised intravenous cannula and attach a cardiac monitor and pulse oximeter to the patient.

(2) Give high-dose, 40–60% oxygen, unless there is a prior history of obstructive airways disease, in which case give 28% oxygen. Aim for an oxygen saturation over 94%.

(3) Give diamorphine 5 mg i.v. for pain with an antiemetic, e.g. metoclopramide 10 mg i.v.

(4) Treat left heart failure:

(i) Sit the patient upright and give a diuretic such as frusemide 40 mg i.v. or twice their usual oral daily dose intravenously, if already on frusemide.

(ii) If not improving, give glyceryl trinitrate (GTN) 300 µg sublingually. Remove the tablet if excessive hypotension (systolic BP less than 100 mmHg) occurs.

(iii) In refractory cases repeat the frusemide and commence a GTN infusion:

    (a) Add GTN 200 mg to 500 ml of 5% dextrose, i.e. 400 µg/ml, using a glass bottle and low absorption polyethylene infusion set.

    (b) Infuse initially at 1 ml/h, maintaining systolic BP above 100 mmHg. Gradually increase to 20 ml/h, avoiding hypotension.

(5) Give low-dose aspirin 150 mg orally unless contraindicated by known hypersensitivity.

(6) If immediate transfer to coronary care is not possible, consider thrombolytic therapy in consultation with the medical team. Aim to commence thrombolysis within a maximum of 30 min of the patient's arrival in hospital.

(i) Thrombolysis is indicated within 12 h of the onset of cardiac pain, in patients with ECG evidence of infarction (ST elevation of at least 1 mm in two contiguous limb leads and 2 mm in two contiguous precordial leads) or bundle branch block, particularly LBBB.

(ii) Absolute contraindications to thrombolysis include:

    (a) Active gastrointestinal bleeding, major surgery or trauma including prolonged CPR in previous 2 weeks.

    (b) Intracerebral or subarachnoid haemorrhage ever.

    (c) Thrombotic stroke in previous 6 months.

    (d) Pregnancy, proliferative diabetic retinopathy, known bleeding diathesis, and uncontrolled hypertension (systolic BP over 200 mmHg, diastolic over 110 mmHg).

    (e) Aortic dissection (see page 19).

(iii) Relative contraindications (thrombolysis may still be considered in those at highest risk of death, or with greatest net clinical benefit, e.g. large anterior infarction presenting early):

    (a) Arterial puncture or central line.

    (b) Past history of gastrointestinal bleeding.

       (c)   Current use of warfarin.

(iv)   Give streptokinase 1.5 million units over 45 min to 1 h in 100 ml normal saline.

       (a)   Continue ECG monitoring throughout for reperfusion arrhythmias.

       (b)   Slow or stop the infusion if hypotension or rash occur. Restart the infusion as soon as they have resolved.

       (c)   Occasionally severe hypotension and anaphylaxis may occur requiring colloids, adrenaline, etc. (see page 107).

(v)   Use alteplase (rt-PA) if the patient has ever had streptokinase before (except within the previous 5 days) or is allergic.

       (a)   Give a bolus of alteplase 15 mg (15 ml), followed by an infusion of 0.75 mg/kg over 30 min (not to exceed 50 mg), then 0.5 mg/kg over 60 min (not to exceed 35 mg).

       (b)   Commence heparin 5000 U i.v. as a bolus, followed by an infusion at 1000 U/h.

(7) Treat cardiac arrhythmias:

   (i)   *Bradycardia*. This may be sinus, junctional (nodal) or due to atrioventricular block:

       (a)   Give a bolus of atropine 0.6 mg i.v.

       (b)   If it persists, repeat the atropine for sinus or junctional bradycardia.

       (c)   If it persists with atrioventricular block, consider inserting a temporary transvenous pacemaker wire. An external (trancutaneous) pacemaker may be used until x-ray guidance is available.

       (d)   Avoid using an isoprenaline infusion, as it may provoke ventricular fibrillation following acute myocardial infarction.

   (ii)   *Ventricular tachycardia (VT)*.

       (a)   If the patient is hypotensive or collapsed, give a 100 J synchronised DC shock, ideally after the anaesthetist has given a short-acting general anaesthetic or intravenous midazolam in the conscious patient.

(b) If the patient is not hypotensive, give ligno-
     caine up to 100 mg i.v. as a bolus and then
     start an infusion of lignocaine at 2–4 mg/min.
(c) If the lignocaine fails, give procainamide 100
     mg slowly i.v., if necessary repeated every 5
     min to a maximum of 17 mg/kg. Then
     continue as an infusion at 2–6 mg/min.

Note: frequent ventricular ectopics do not require treatment,
unless they are multifocal or arrive on the T wave of the
preceding complex.

(iii) *Supraventricular tachycardia.*
       (a) If the patient is shocked or hypotensive,
            proceed directly to synchronised DC cardio-
            version starting at 100 J after the anaesthetist
            has given a short acting anaesthetic.
       (b) In the absence of shock, continue oxygen and
            check that pain, anxiety or heart failure have
            been treated.
       (c) Then use a vagal stimulus such as carotid
            sinus massage: press firmly at the upper
            border of the thyroid cartilage against the
            vertebral process with a circular motion.
       (d) If this fails, give verapamil 5–10 mg i.v. as a
            bolus over 30 s to 2 min. Verapamil may
            cause hypotension and bradycardia, particu-
            larly in elderly patients, who should be
            pretreated with calcium gluconate 10 ml
            given slowly i.v.
       (e) Never use verapamil after a beta blocker, or if
            digitalis toxicity is suspected or the patient
            has a wide complex tachycardia (see below).
       (f) Alternatively, use adenosine particularly in
            wide complex tachycardia, which may either
            be due to supraventricular tachycardia with
            aberrant conduction or ventricular tachy-
            cardia.
       (g) Give adenosine 3 mg rapidly over 2 s i.v.,
            followed by 6 mg rapidly after 1–2 min, then 12
            mg rapidly if still no response. Transient facial

flushing, dyspnoea, chest pressure and nausea may occur. Give a reduced initial dose of 1 mg if the patient is on dipyridamole. Persistence of the arrhythmia suggests VT, thus treat as in (7)(ii).

(iv) *Atrial flutter and fibrillation.*

    (a) If the patient is shocked or hypotensive, proceed directly to synchronised DC cardioversion starting at 50 J. In patients on digoxin therapy, a temporary transvenous pacemaker may be required as asystole may follow DC shock.

    (b) Otherwise, give verapamil 5–10 mg i.v. to slow the ventricular rate. This is followed by digitalising the patient with digoxin 500 µg orally or slowly intravenously.

    (c) Alternatively give amiodarone 5 mg/kg diluted in 250 ml of 5% dextrose over 30 min to achieve sinus rhythm. Beware precipitating bradycardia in patients already on beta blockers, calcium antagonists or digoxin.

(8) Refer the patient immediately to the medical team for admission to the coronary care unit, if they are not already involved.

Note: the ECG may be normal, and the patient deceptively well after a myocardial infarction. Take note of any preceding episode of sweating, nausea, vomiting or collapse and refer the patient to the medical team if you have any clinical suspicions of cardiac infarction.

PULMONARY EMBOLUS (PE)

DIAGNOSIS

(1) Predisposing factors include pre-existing cardiovascular or respiratory disease, cancer, DVT or previous thromboembolism, immobilisation, trauma or recent surgery, pregnancy and the oral contraceptive pill.

(2) A small PE causes pleuritic pain and possibly haemoptysis, with few physical signs; but look for a low-grade

pyrexia (37.5°C), tachypnoea, tachycardia and a pleural rub.

(3) A major PE causes dyspnoea and sudden collapse, with cyanosis, tachycardia, hypotension, a parasternal heave, raised JVP and a loud delayed pulmonary second sound.

(4) The CXR may be normal or show a blunted costophrenic angle, raised hemidiaphragm, an area of infarction or linear atelectasis, or an area of oligaemia.

(5) The ECG may show a tachycardia only or possibly right axis deviation, right heart strain, RBBB and atrial fibrillation.

(6) Blood gases will reflect hypoxia and hypocapnia from hyperventilation, but may be normal.

MANAGEMENT

(1) Establish venous access with a heparinised intravenous cannula and attach a cardiac monitor and pulse oximeter to the patient.

(2) Give high-dose oxygen through a face mask. Aim for an oxygen saturation above 94%.

(3) Relieve pain if it is severe with diamorphine 5 mg i.v. and give an antiemetic such as metoclopramide 10 mg i.v.

(4) Commence heparin 5000 U i.v. as a bolus, followed by 1000 U/h in the high-probability patient without contraindications.

(5) Refer the patient to the medical team for a ventilation-perfusion lung scan or pulmonary angiography if available.

AORTIC DISSECTION

DIAGNOSIS

(1) Predisposed to by hypertension, Marfan's syndrome or trauma.

(2) The pain is sudden, tearing, retrosternal or in the back, migratory, and may be severe and resistant to opiates.

(3) Look for absent pulses, a difference of blood pressure in the arms, or the complications of the dissection:

    (i)   myocardial ischaemia, aortic incompetence and haemopericardium with pericardial rub or cardiac tamponade (see page 10);

    (ii)   pleural rub or effusion;

    (iii) altered consciousness, hemiplegia or paraplegia;

    (iv) oliguria and haematuria;

    (v)   intestinal ischaemia or bowel infarction.

(4) The CXR may show a widened mediastinum, blurred aortic knob and a left pleural effusion.

(5) The ECG remains remarkably normal despite the severity of the pain, but often shows left ventricular hypertrophy.

MANAGEMENT

(1) Establish venous access with a large-bore (14- or 16-gauge) heparinised intravenous cannula, send blood for group and cross-match, and attach a cardiac monitor and pulse oximeter to the patient.

(2) Give high-dose oxygen via a face mask. Aim for an oxygen saturation above 94%.

(3) Relieve the pain with diamorphine 5 mg i.v. and give an antiemetic.

(4) Reduce the systolic BP to below 110 mmHg using a labetalol infusion, or sodium nitroprusside plus propranolol in consultation with the medical team.

(5) Refer the patient for urgent transoesophageal echocardiography, CT scan or aortography to confirm the diagnosis. Contact the cardiothoracic surgeons.

PERICARDITIS

DIAGNOSIS

(1) This may be postviral or follow a myocardial infarction, pericardiotomy, connective tissue disorder, uraemia, trauma, tuberculosis and a neoplasm.

(2) The pain is sharp, pleuritic, retrosternal and relieved by sitting forward.

(3) A pericardial friction rub is best heard along the left sternal edge with the patient sitting forward, and is usually present at some stage.

(4) An ECG may show tachycardia alone, widespread concave ST elevation or atrial fibrillation.

(5) The CXR is usually normal, even if a pericardial effusion is present.

MANAGEMENT

(1) Give the patient a nonsteroidal anti-inflammatory agent such as diclofenac (Voltarol) 50 mg orally t.d.s. or ibuprofen 400 mg orally t.d.s.

(2) Send blood for FBC, U&E, cardiac enzymes and viral serology.

(3) Refer the patient to the medical team for cardiac monitoring. Echocardiography and pericardiocentesis are indicated for signs of cardiac tamponade such as tachycardia, hypotension, pulsus paradoxus and a raised JVP that rises on inspiration — known as Kussmaul's sign (see page 10).

PLEURISY

DIAGNOSIS

(1) Pleurisy or pleuritic pain occurs in association with pneumonia, pulmonary infarction, neoplasia, TB, connective tissue disorders, uraemia and following trauma.

(2) It may also be due to viruses especially enteroviruses, and be mimicked by a pneumothorax or epidemic myalgia (Bornholm disease).

(3) The pain is sharp, localised and exacerbated by moving, coughing or breathing, which tends to be shallow. Radiation to the shoulder or abdomen occurs with diaphragmatic involvement.

(4) A pleural rub is heard, although it may be inaudible if pain limits deep breathing, and disappears as an effusion develops.

(5) The CXR may reveal the underlying cause or be quite normal.

MANAGEMENT

(1) Give the patient oxygen and a nonsteroidal anti-inflammatory agent such as diclofenac (Voltarol) 50 mg orally t.d.s. or ibuprofen 400 mg orally t.d.s.
(2) Send arterial blood gases if there are significant signs of pulmonary parenchymal disease and perform an ECG.
(3) Refer the patient to the medical team for treatment of the underlying cause or to exclude a pulmonary embolus, which is possible despite a normal CXR and ECG (see page 18).

PNEUMONIA

DIAGNOSIS

(1) Fever, dyspnoea, productive cough, haemoptysis and pleuritic chest pain are present.
(2) Examination may reveal signs of lobar infection, with a dull percussion note and bronchial breathing, but usually there are only localised moist crepitations with diminished breath sounds.
(3) The CXR shows diffuse shadowing unless there is lobar consolidation.

MANAGEMENT

(1) Give the patient high-dose oxygen, unless there is a known history of obstructive airways disease (use 28%). Aim for an oxygen saturation above 94%.
(2) Take blood for blood culture, WCC, U&E and blood sugar. Check the blood gases.
(3) Commence benzylpenicillin 1 Mu (600 mg) i.v. or erythromycin 500 mg orally if atypical pneumonia is suspected, and refer the patient to the medical team.
(4) Young, fit adults with single lobe involvement may be well enough to return home on amoxycillin 500 mg

orally t.d.s. or erythromycin 500 mg orally q.d.s. both for 5 days. Inform the general practitioner by telephone or a letter, if the patient is not admitted.

PNEUMOTHORAX

DIAGNOSIS

(1) This may occur spontaneously (especially in Marfan's syndrome or in tall, asthenic body types), from trauma and in association with chronic lung disease, e.g. asthma, emphysema and cystic fibrosis.
(2) It may only cause slight dyspnoea and pleuritic chest pain, even when the whole lung is collapsed. Significant dyspnoea with loss of usual exercise tolerance is common in chronic lung disease.
(3) Examination shows reduced chest expansion on the affected side, increased resonance on percussion and diminished breath sounds.
(4) Request a CXR on inspiration and expiration in all cases. Do not wait for this if there are signs of tension, but proceed immediately to insertion of a wide-bore cannula or intercostal drain (see page 10).

MANAGEMENT

(1) Patients with a small to moderate (lung collapsed less than halfway to heart border) pneumothorax and with no significant dyspnoea and no chronic lung disease may go home.[3]
  (i)   Arrange immediate follow-up with the general practitioner and medical outpatients in one week. Advise against air travel until changes on the CXR have resolved.
(2) Simple aspiration is appropriate for patients without chronic lung disease, with complete collapse or significant dyspnoea:
  (i)   Infiltrate local anaesthetic down to the pleura in the second intercostal space in the mid-clavicular line.

    (ii)   Insert a 16-gauge cannula into the pleural cavity, withdraw the needle and connect to a 50 ml syringe with three-way tap.

    (iii)   Aspirate air until resistance is felt, the patient coughs excessively or more than 2500 ml are aspirated.

    (iv)   Repeat the CXR and refer the patient to the medical team for overnight admission.

(3) Otherwise, an intercostal drain is indicated for:

    (i)   Tension pneumothorax.

    (ii)   Traumatic pneumothorax or haemothorax.

    (iii)   A pneumothorax causing significant dyspnoea, if there is pre-existing chronic lung disease.

    (iv)   Any pneumothorax prior to anaesthesia or positive pressure ventilation.

    (v)   Failed simple aspiration, e.g. more than just a small residual rim of air around the lung.

(4) Insertion of an intercostal drain:

    (i)   Insert the drain into the fifth intercostal space in the midaxillary line, after infiltration with local anaesthetic down to the pleura.

    (ii)   Use a scalpel blade to incise the skin and subcutaneous fat, followed by blunt dissection down to and through the parietal pleura.

    (iii)   Slide the drain in gently without any forcible use of the trocar.

    (iv)   Use a size 20–24 French gauge directed apically for a simple pneumothorax, or a larger 28–32 French gauge directed basally for a haemothorax. Connect the drain to an underwater seal.

ABDOMINAL CAUSES OF CHEST PAIN

DIAGNOSIS AND MANAGEMENT

(1) *Oesophagitis*.

    (i)   This is suggested by burning retrosternal or epigastric pain, worse on stooping, exacerbated by hot drinks or food and relieved by antacids.

    (ii)   It may mimic cardiac pain and be relieved by sublingual glyceryl trinitrate, so refer the patient to the medical team if there is doubt about the diagnosis, even if the ECG is normal.

(iii) Otherwise give an antacid and metoclopramide 5 mg orally t.d.s.

(2) *Oesophageal rupture.* See page 155 in the chapter on chest injuries.

(3) *Acute cholecystitis, pancreatitis* and *peptic ulceration* can cause chest pain, but other diagnostic features should be present.

MUSCULOSKELETAL AND CHEST WALL PAIN

DIAGNOSIS AND MANAGEMENT

(1) Musculoskeletal disorders cause pain that is worse with movement and breathing. There may have been preceding strenuous exercise, a bout of coughing or a history of minor trauma.

(2) Pain is localised on palpation and the ECG is normal. A CXR may show a fractured rib but is otherwise normal.

(3) Give the patient a nonsteroidal anti-inflammatory analgesic such as diclofenac 50 mg orally t.d.s. or ibuprofen 400 mg orally t.d.s. and refer back to the general practitioner.

(4) Two specific causes are:

(i) *Costochondritis: Tietze's syndrome.* This causes localised pain and tenderness typically around the second costochondral junction.

(a) Prescribe diclofenac 50 mg orally t.d.s. or ibuprofen 400 mg orally t.d.s. and refer the patient back to the general practitioner.

(ii) *Shingles.* Shingles causes pain localised to a dermatome, unaffected by breathing, associated with an area of hyperaesthesia preceding the characteristic rash.

(a) Give the patient, usually elderly, with severe pain a narcotic analgesic and acyclovir 800 mg orally five times a day, if seen within 72 h of vesicle eruption.

(b) Admit to a suitable isolation area if unable to be nursed at home.

THE BREATHLESS PATIENT

DIFFERENTIAL DIAGNOSIS

The causes to consider include the following, some of which were covered in the preceding chapter on chest pain:

(1) acute asthma;
(2) pulmonary oedema;
(3) pulmonary embolus;
(4) pneumonia and exacerbation of bronchitis;
(5) pneumothorax;
(6) acute upper airway obstruction;
(7) metabolic causes such as acidosis in diabetic ketosis or salicylate poisoning;
(8) muscular weakness from myasthenia gravis or Guillain–Barré syndrome.

ACUTE ASTHMA

DIAGNOSIS

(1) Ascertain the precipitating factors in the present attack, its duration, treatment given including steroids and theophylline derivatives and the response to treatment.
(2) Ask about previous attacks, hospital admissions, ventilation in an intensive care unit and the regular use of steroids.
(3) The highest-risk categories for a severe attack are:
  (i)   The 'morning dipper' — the patient who wakes breathless in the early morning.
  (ii) A recent acute attack within the last month, especially if the patient required steroids.
  (iii) The 'brittle' asthmatic prone to sudden catastrophic attacks.
(4) To assess the severity of the present attack, carefully examine the patient *before* any nebuliser therapy is given. A severe attack is indicated by any of the following:[4]
  (i)   inability to complete sentences in one breath:
  (ii) respiratory rate 25 or more breaths per minute;

    (iii)   tachycardia 110 or more beats per minute;
    (iv)   peak expiratory flow (PEF) 50% or less of pre-
             dicted or best (see Fig. 2).
(5) A life-threatening attack is indicated by any of the
    following:[4]
    (i)   PEF under 33% of predicted or best;
    (ii)   silent chest, cyanosis or feeble respiratory effort;
    (iii)   bradycardia or hypotension;
    (iv)   exhaustion, confusion or coma.

MANAGEMENT

(1) Commence high-dose oxygen via a face mask. Maintain
    the oxygen saturation above 92%.

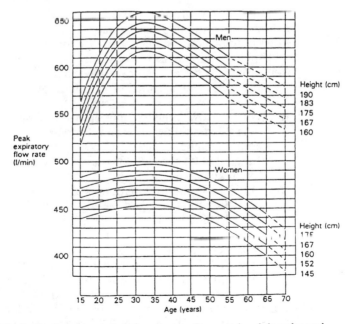

Fig. 2. Predicted normal peak expiratory flow rate in adult males and females. (Reproduced by kind permission of *Clement Clarke International Ltd.*)

(2) Give salbutamol 5 mg via an oxygen-driven nebuliser, diluted with 3 ml normal saline.

(3) If there is no response, or a life-threatening attack, add ipratropium (Atrovent) 500 µg to a second dose of salbutamol 5 mg via the nebuliser.

(4) If the patient is still wheezy, refer to the medical team for admission and perform the following:

    (i)   Arterial blood gases. Markers of a very severe, life-threatening attack are:

        (a) Normal (5–6 kPa) or high $PaCO_2$;

        (b) Severe hypoxia — PaO_2 under 8 kPa;

        (c) A low pH (or high hydrogen ion concentration).

    (ii)   A CXR to look for a pneumothorax or an area of consolidation.

    (iii) Send blood for WCC, U&E, blood sugar and commence an intravenous infusion of normal saline if the patient is dehydrated.

    (iv) Give prednisolone 50 mg orally or hydrocortisone 200 mg i.v. if unable to swallow. Repeat the salbutamol 5 mg via the nebuliser up to every 15–30 min.

    (v)   Commence an intravenous bronchodilator under ECG control:

        (a) Give a slow bolus of aminophylline 5 mg/kg over 20 min followed by an infusion of 500 mg aminophylline in 500 ml of 5% dextrose, i.e. 1 mg/ml at 0.5 mg/kg/h (35 ml/h or 0.58 ml/min for 70-kg patient).

        (b) Omit the bolus if the patient is already taking oral theophylline and send blood for a theophylline level.

        (c) Or omit the aminophylline altogether and give salbutamol 250 µg i.v. over 10 min instead, followed by an infusion of 5 mg salbutamol in 500 ml of 5% dextrose, i.e. 10 µg/ml at 5 µg/min (30 ml/h or 0.5 ml/min) initially.

    (vi) Call the anaesthetist for a deteriorating patient with hypoxia (PaO_2 less than 8 kPa), hypercapnia ($PaCO_2$ over 6 kPa) or any features of a life-threatening attack and admit to the intensive care unit.

(5) Meanwhile, in the patient with a mild attack (PEF over 75% predicted) or moderate attack (PEF 50–75% predicted) that improves with nebuliser therapy alone to a PEF over 75%:

    (i) Discharge if the general practitioner can provide early follow-up and the patient has salbutamol and beclomethasone inhalers (and knows how to use them), and prednisolone 50 mg orally daily reduced over 7 days.

    (ii) If there is any doubt about discharging the patient, refer to the medical team for their opinion first.

PULMONARY OEDEMA

DIAGNOSIS

(1) Pulmonary ocdema is usually caused by left ventricular failure due to myocardial infarction, hypertension, an arrhythmia, fluid overload or valvular disease.

(2) Occasional noncardiac causes include septicaemia, uraemia, head injury and inhalation of smoke or noxious gases.

(3) The patient is clammy, distressed, preferring to sit upright, and may have a tachycardia, basal crepitations and a triple rhythm.

(4) The CXR shows engorged upper-lobe veins, a perihilar haze, cardiomegaly, septal Kerley B lines and bilateral pleural effusions.

(5) The ECG may help indicate the aetiology.

MANAGEMENT

(1) Sit the patient upright and give 40–60% oxygen, unless the patient is known to have chronic bronchitis when 28% oxygen should be used. Aim for an oxygen saturation above 94%.

(2) Give frusemide 40 mg i.v. or twice their usual oral daily dose i.v., if already on frusemide.

(3) Give morphine 1–2.5 mg i.v. with an antiemetic such as metoclopramide 10 mg i.v.

(4) If not improving, give glyceryl trinitrate 300 µg sublingually. Remove the tablet if excessive hypotension (systolic BP less than 100 mmHg) occurs.

(5) In refractory cases repeat the frusemide and commence a glyceryl trinitrate (GTN) infusion:

  (i)   Add GTN 200 mg to 500 ml of 5% dextrose, i.e. 400 µg/ml, using a glass bottle and low absorption polyethylene infusion set.

  (ii) Infuse initially at 1 ml/h, maintaining systolic BP above 100 mmHg. Gradually increase to 20 ml/h, avoiding hypotension.

(6) Refer the patient immediately to the medical team.

Note: if the patient has chronic obstructive airways disease or asthma do not give the morphine.

PULMONARY EMBOLUS

See page 18.

PNEUMONIA

See page 22.

PNEUMOTHORAX

See page 23.

ACUTE UPPER AIRWAY OBSTRUCTION

DIAGNOSIS

(1) Acute upper airway obstruction may be due to croup, epiglottitis, inhaled foreign body, smoke inhalation, angioneurotic oedema, trauma, carcinoma or retropharyngeal abscess.

(2) There is severe distress, ineffective respiratory efforts, stridor and cyanosis followed by unconsciousness. There may also be hoarseness, or complete aphonia.

MANAGEMENT

This depends on the suspected cause.

(1) Sit the patient up and give 100% oxygen via a face mask. Attach a cardiac monitor and pulse oximeter to the patient. Aim for an oxygen saturation above 94%.

(2) If inhalation of a foreign body is suspected:

  (i) Perform the Heimlich manoeuvre. Stand behind the patient, place your arms around the upper abdomen with your hands clasped in the epigastrium and give thrusts upwards to expel the obstruction.

  (ii) Hold an infant or small child head-down instead and deliver five back blows with the heel of the free hand.

  (iii) If the foreign body is still present, attempt removal under direct vision using a laryngoscope and a pair of long-handled Magill forceps.

  (iv) If the patient is *in extremis* and all else has failed, proceed to cricothyrotomy (see Fig. 3):

     (a) Extend the patient's neck and identify the cricothyroid membrane between the lower border of the thyroid cartilage and the upper border of the cricoid cartilage.

     (b) Achieve rapid access by inserting a large-bore 14-gauge intravenous cannula through the cricothyroid membrane.

     (c) Attach this to wall oxygen at 15 l/min using a Y-connector. Insufflate oxygen by intermittent occlusion of the open end of the Y-connector for 1 second in every 5.

     (d) Alternatively make an incision through the cricothyroid membrane with a scalpel blade, and insert a 4–6 mm ET tube (or small tracheostomy tube) and connect this to an Ambu or Laerdal bag and the oxygen supply.

(3) *Croup* (see page 279). A child with croup will have a barking cough, harsh stridor, hoarseness and be frightened and miserable but not systemically ill. Refer to the paediatric team.

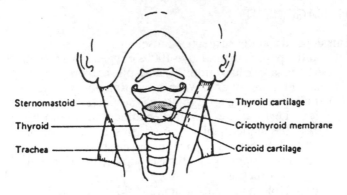

Sternomastoid ——

Thyroid ——

Trachea ——

—— Thyroid cartilage

—— Cricothyroid membrane

—— Cricoid cartilage

(a)

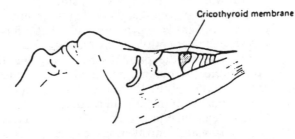

Cricothyroid membrane

(b)

Fig. 3. Cricothyrotomy. The anatomical relationship of the cricothyroid membrane are shown: (a) AP view; (b) oblique lateral view.

(4) *Epiglottitis* (see page 280). Inflammation of the epiglottis presents with sudden onset of difficulty in breathing, soft inspiratory stridor, dysphagia and drooling. The child looks toxic and unwell.

    (i)   Do not examine further — i.e. no rectal temperature, BP, nor x-ray. Do not attempt to visualise the throat.

    (ii)   Leave the parent holding the child upright with an oxygen mask held near the child's face.

(iii) Call for senior paediatric, anaesthetic and ENT assistance immediately.

(5) *Smoke inhalation* (see page 169). This requires:
    (i) 100% oxygen, nebulised salbutamol and referral to the medical team or specialist burns unit if there is an associated respiratory burn. Be prepared to intubate if gross laryngeal oedema occurs.
    (ii) Send blood for blood gases and a carboxyhaemo-globin level.

(6) *Angioneurotic oedema* (see page 106). This condition requires:
    (i) High-dose oxygen and 0.3–0.5 ml of 1 in 1000 adrenaline intramuscularly, repeated as necessary, or 0.75–1.5 µg/kg i.e. 50–100 µg or 0.5–1.0 ml of 1 in 10 000 adrenaline for a 70-kg patient given slowly i.v. if circulatory collapse occurs.
    (ii) Chlorpheniramine 10 mg i.v. plays a secondary role to adrenaline in severe cases.
    (iii) Intubation may still be required, ideally performed by a skilled anaesthetist.

UPPER GASTROINTESTINAL HAEMORRHAGE

DIAGNOSIS

(1) This presents as:
    (i) haematemesis and/or melaena;
    (ii) haematochezia — bright red rectal bleeding;
    (iii) collapse and shock;
    (iv) syncope and postural hypotension;
    (v) fatigue, dyspnoea, angina, etc.

(2) Causes include:
    (i) peptic ulceration (over 50% of cases);
    (ii) gastritis:
        (a) post-alcohol;
        (b) drug-induced (salicylates, nonsteroidal anti-inflammatory drugs);

(iii)   Mallory–Weiss tear — oesophageal tear following vomiting or retching;

(iv)   bleeding oesophageal or gastric varices associated with portal hypertension (usually due to alcoholic cirrhosis);

(v)   reflux oesophagitis;

(vi)   others including gastric neoplasm, blood coagulation disorders, or a connective tissue disorder.

MANAGEMENT

(1) If the patient is shocked, give oxygen and attach a pulse oximeter and cardiac monitor to the patient. Establish venous access with a large-bore 14-gauge intravenous cannula.

(2) (i)   Take blood for Hb, PCV, U&E, blood sugar and cross-match from 2 to 4 units of blood, according to the presumed aetiology and degree of shock.

(ii)   If liver disease is suspected, check the LFTs and clotting studies including a PTI. Examine for jaundice, bruising, gynaecomastia, spider naevi, palmar erythema, clubbing, hepatomegaly and encephalopathy. If portal hypertension is suspected, examine for splenomegaly and ascites.

(iii)   As transfusion will preclude further investigation, take blood for later vitamin B_{12} and folate levels.

(3) Commence a transfusion:

(i)   ideally with cross-matched blood when it is available;

(ii)   pending this, if the patient is shocked, use plasma, polygeline (Haemaccel), or O-negative blood if the situation is desperate;

(iii)   otherwise use normal saline.

(4) Arrange for an urgent endoscopy, particularly in patients who continue to bleed, have suspected varices or are aged over 60 years.

(i)   Endoscopy will differentiate the cause of the bleeding and allow immediate thermal or injection therapy where appropriate.

(5) Refer every case to the medical team for admission. A surgical opinion is indicated if endoscopic therapy fails or is unavailable.

Note: inserting a CVP line in a hypotensive, shocked patient is difficult and dangerous and is best left until initial transfusion is underway for the anaesthetist or another skilled doctor to perform.

DIABETIC COMA AND PRE-COMA

Hypoglycaemia rapidly produces coma in diabetics, compared with the slower onset of altered consciousness in diabetic ketoacidosis and hyperosmolar nonketotic coma.

DIABETIC KETOACIDOSIS (DKA)

DIAGNOSIS

(1) This condition may occur in a known diabetic, precipitated by trauma, infection, myocardial infarction, cerebral infarction or inadequate insulin therapy (e.g. insulin stopped in an unwell diabetic patient 'because he is not eating').

(2) Alternatively, it may arise *de novo* in an undiagnosed diabetic, heralded by polyuria, polydipsia, weight loss, abdominal pain, lethargy or coma.

(3) The predominant features arise from salt and water depletion and acidosis; hence there is dry skin, tachycardia, hypotension (especially postural) and deep sighing respirations (Kussmaul breathing).

   (i)   The ketones may be detected on the breath as a sickly sweet smell.

Note: every patient who presents with abdominal pain, vomiting or thirst must have urine tested for sugar and ketones.

MANAGEMENT

(1) Attach a cardiac monitor and pulse oximeter to the patient, give oxygen and aim for an oxygen saturation above 94%.

(2) Establish venous access and send blood urgently for U&E and blood sugar, blood cultures and FBC.

(3) Start an intravenous infusion and run in 500 ml normal saline, followed by a further 1000 ml in the next hour, if the diagnosis is confirmed.

(4) Send blood for blood gases and organise a CXR, ECG and MSU.

(5) If the patient is unconscious, pass a nasogastric tube and catheterise the bladder.

(6) (i)   Give soluble insulin 10 U i.v. stat.
    (ii) Commence an insulin infusion: add 50 U soluble insulin to 500 ml Haemaccel, i.e. 1 U/10 ml, and run at 5 U/h or 50 ml/h.
    (iii) Continue the intravenous normal saline resuscitation which is of equal importance to the insulin.

(7) Add potassium (K) to the intravenous fluid when the plasma potassium level is known (this should be within 30 min).
    (i)   If K is less than 3.0 mmol/l, give 40 mmol KCl/h (3 g KCl).
    (ii) If K is 3.0–4.0 mmol/l, give 26.8 mmol KCl/h (2 g KCl).
    (iii) If K is 4.0–5.0 mmol/l, give 20 mmol KCl/h (1.5 g KCl).
    (iv) If K is 5.0–6.0 mmol/l, give 13.4 mmol KCl/h (1 g KCl).
    (v)   Stop the potassium if:
          (a) the patient is anuric;
          (b) the level is over 6.0 mmol/l;
          (c) the ECG shows peaked T waves or QRS complex widening.

(8) Refer the patient immediately to the medical team.

(9) Do not give intravenous sodium bicarbonate except on the advice of the diabetic team. It may be considered if the pH remains below 7.0 with incipient circulatory failure.

HYPEROSMOLAR NONKETOTIC COMA

DIAGNOSIS

(1) Hyperosmolar nonketotic coma is more common in the elderly, non-insulin-dependent patient.

(2) It is precipitated by thiazide diuretic use or infection, myocardial infarction or a stroke.

(3) The patient presents with an altered level of consciousness and focal neurological signs. Mortality is 50%.

(4) Blood glucose and serum osmolarity tend to be higher than in DKA. Osmolarity usually exceeds 350 mosmol/l.
    (i) It may be estimated by 2(Na + K) + urea + glucose (all units in mmol/l).

MANAGEMENT

(1) This is comparable to DKA (see page 35).

(2) Give intravenous normal saline, or half-normal saline if the serum sodium exceeds 150 mmol/l.

(3) Lower insulin and initial potassium replacement rates are needed than in DKA.

(4) Commence a prophylactic heparin infusion at 1000 U/h.

ACID–BASE AND ELECTROLYTE DISTURBANCES

Metabolic or respiratory acidosis or alkalosis and hypokalaemia or hyperkalaemia may all present as life-threatening emergencies, sometimes with minimal preceding clinical features.

METABOLIC ACIDOSIS

DIAGNOSIS

(1) Causes may either be associated with an increased anion gap over 15, calculated from Na + K – (Cl + HCO_3), all units in mmol/l. These include:

(i)   Increased acid production:
   (a) Ketoacidosis e.g. diabetic, alcoholic, starvation.
   (b) Lactic acidosis e.g. cardiac arrest, shock, hypoxia and anaemia or liver failure, sepsis, pancreatitis and drugs such as phenformin.
(ii)   Exogenous acid ingestion:
   (a) salicylate;
   (b) methanol;
   (c) ethylene glycol.
(iii) Decreased acid excretion:
   (a) renal failure.

(2) Or causes may be associated with a normal anion gap under 15. The loss of bicarbonate is balanced by an increase in chloride resulting in hyperchloraemia. These include:

(i)   Loss of alkali:
   (a) diarrhoea;
   (b) small bowel fistula;
   (c) ureterosigmoidostomy;
   (d) carbonic anhydrase inhibitors.
(ii)   Decreased hydrogen ion excretion:
   (a) hyperaldosteronism;
   (b) distal renal tubular acidosis.
(iii) Administration of cationic acids:
   (a) synthetic amino acid solutions;
   (b) ammonium chloride.

(3) There is a primary fall in plasma bicarbonate below 22 mmol/l.

Table 4. Primary acid–base disturbances with expected compensatory response

Disorder	Primary change	Compensatory response
Metabolic acidosis	↓ bicarbonate	Rapid ↓ $PaCO_2$
Metabolic alkalosis	↑ bicarbonate	Variable ↑ $PaCO_2$
Respiratory acidosis:		
Acute	↑ $PaCO_2$	Immediate, small ↑ bicarbonate
Chronic	↑ $PaCO_2$	Slow, larger ↑ bicarbonate
Respiratory alkalosis:		
Acute	↓ $PaCO_2$	Immediate ↓ bicarbonate
Chronic	↓ $PaCO_2$	Slow, larger ↓ bicarbonate

(4) There is a compensatory fall in the $PaCO_2$ (see Table 4).
  (i)   Predicted $PaCO_2$ (mmHg) = 1.25 HCO_3 (mmol/l) + 10.
  (ii) To convert predicted $PaCO_2$ in mmHg to kPa, multiply by 0.133.
(5) There are few specific clinical features in acute metabolic acidosis other than hyperventilation.

MANAGEMENT

(1) Give oxygen and commence intravenous fluid to maintain the circulation.
(2) Correct any reversible underlying disorder such as diabetic ketoacidosis.
(3) Refer the patient to the medical team. Dialysis will be necessary for renal failure, and severe salicylate or methanol poisoning.

METABOLIC ALKALOSIS

DIAGNOSIS

(1) Causes are due to a loss of hydrogen ion or a gain of bicarbonate, usually in association with an extracellular fluid deficit, hyperaldosteronism or severe hypokalaemia:
  (i)   Loss of hydrogen ion:
        (a) vomiting, gastric aspiration;
        (b) diuretics, steroids, carbenoxolone;
        (c) Cushing's, Conn's, Bartter's syndromes.
  (ii) Gain of bicarbonate:
        (a) excess bicarbonate including antacids;
        (b) metabolism of lactate, citrate, acetate.
(2) There is a primary increase in plasma bicarbonate above 28 mmol/l.
(3) There is a compensatory rise in $PaCO_2$ (see Table 4).
  (i)   Predicted $PaCO_2$ (mmHg) = $\dfrac{HCO_3 (mmol/l)}{2}$ + 30.
  (ii) To convert predicted $PaCO_2$ in mmHg to kPa, multiply by 0.133.

(4) There are no specific clinical features.

MANAGEMENT

(1) Correct any reversible underlying disorder.
(2) Give normal saline i.v. with potassium if low.

RESPIRATORY ACIDOSIS

DIAGNOSIS

(1) Causes are due to ventilatory failure:
    (i)   Acute ventilatory failure:
        (a) sedative drugs e.g. opiates, barbiturates, benzodiazepines;
        (b) head injury, thoracic trauma;
        (c) stroke;
        (d) neuromuscular disorders e.g. Guillain–Barré, myasthenia gravis.
    (ii)   Chronic ventilatory failure:
        (a) chronic obstructive pulmonary disease;
        (b) marked obesity.
(2) There is a primary increase in $PaCO_2$ above 44 mmHg.
(3) There is a compensatory rise in plasma bicarbonate (see Table 4).
    (i)   To convert $PaCO_2$ in kPa to mmHg, multiply by 7.518.
    (ii)   In acute respiratory acidosis, predicted HCO_3 (mmol/l)
$$= \frac{PaCO_2(mmHg)}{10} + 20.$$
    (iii)   In chronic respiratory acidosis, predicted HCO_3 (mmol/l)
$$= \frac{PaCO_2(mmHg)}{2} + 2.$$
(4) Hypercapnia leads to confusion, coma and a bounding pulse, although associated hypoxia may dominate the clinical picture.

MANAGEMENT

(1) Give oxygen and commence assisted ventilation by bag-mask ventilation or endotracheal intubation.

(2) Correct any reversible underlying disorder e.g. naloxone for opiate poisoning.

(3) Remember that the pulse oximeter may record a normal oxygen saturation in a patient receiving supplemental oxygen, despite the presence of dangerous hypoventilation.

RESPIRATORY ALKALOSIS

DIAGNOSIS

(1) Causes include:
- (i)   Hypoxia:
    - (a) acute e.g. asthma, pneumonia, pulmonary oedema;
    - (b) chronic e.g. pulmonary fibrosis, altitude, anaemia.
- (ii) Respiratory centre stimulation:
    - (a) fever, thyrotoxicosis;
    - (b) head injury, CNS disease;
    - (c) salicylate poisoning;
    - (d) pain, fear, anxiety;
    - (e) pregnancy;
    - (f) sympathomimetics.
- (iii) Excessive artificial ventilation.

(2) There is a primary decrease in $PaCO_2$ below 36 mmHg.

(3) There is a compensatory fall in plasma bicarbonate (see Table 4).
- (i)   To convert $PaCO_2$ in kPa to mmHg, multiply by 7.518.
- (ii) In acute respiratory alkalosis, predicted HCO_3 (mmol/l)
$$= \frac{PaCO_2(mmHg)}{4} + 14.$$
- (iii) In chronic respiratory alkalosis, predicted HCO_3 (mmol/l)

$$= \frac{PaCO_2(mmHg)}{2} + 4.$$

(4) Light-headedness, paraesthesiae, tingling and numbness with tetany occur.

MANAGEMENT

(1) Look for and correct any reversible underlying disorder.
(2) Never diagnose hysterical hyperventilation until subtle presentations of pneumonia, PE, pneumothorax, fever, etc. have been excluded.
   (i)   Reassure the patient and ask them to rebreathe into a paper bag, if hyperventilation is likely.

HYPOKALAEMIA

DIAGNOSIS

(1) Causes include:
   (i)   Inadequate intake e.g. alcoholism, starvation.
   (ii)   Abnormal GI losses:
          (a) vomiting, diarrhoea.
   (iii) Abnormal renal losses:
          (a) Cushing's, Conn's, Bartter's syndromes;
          (b) ectopic ACTH production;
          (c) drugs e.g. diuretics, steroids, carbenoxolone;
          (d) hypomagnesaemia.
   (iv)   Compartmental shift:
          (a) alkalosis;
          (b) insulin;
          (c) salbutamol, terbutaline, aminophylline.
(2) Weakness, lassitude, paralytic ileus and eventually thirst and polyuria occur.
(3) Nonspecific ECG changes include:
   (i)   T wave inversion, prominent U waves;
   (ii)   Prolonged QT interval;
   (iii) Ventricular arrhythmias including *torsades de pointes*.

MANAGEMENT

(1) Attach an ECG monitor, gain intravenous access and replace potassium immediately in the following:
   (i)   Serum potassium below 3.0 mmol/l;
   (ii) Serum potassium 3.0–3.5 mmol/l in patients in chronic heart failure or with cardiac arrhythmias particularly if on digoxin or following myocardial infarction.
(2) Give potassium 10–20 mmol/h i.v. (never exceed 40 mmol/h) under ECG control.
(3) Change to oral supplements or maintenance intravenous replacement when the serum potassium is above 3.5 mmol/l.
(4) Refer the patient to the medical team.

HYPERKALAEMIA

DIAGNOSIS

(1) Causes include:
   (i)   Spurious e.g. haemolysed specimen, thrombocytosis.
   (ii) Excessive exogenous or endogenous intake:
       (a) potassium supplements, blood transfusion;
       (b) rhabdomyolysis, burns.
   (iii) Decreased excretion:
       (a) renal failure, Addison's disease;
       (b) drugs e.g. potassium-sparing diuretics, ACE inhibitors, NSAIDs.
   (iv) Compartmental shift:
       (a) acidosis;
       (b) digoxin poisoning, suxamethonium.
(2) Weakness, flaccid paralysis and paraesthesiae occur.
(3) ECG changes are characteristic:
   (i)   Peaked T waves;
   (ii) ST depression, prolonged PR interval;
   (iii) QRS widening, absent P waves, sine wave pattern;
   (iv) Ventricular tachycardia, fibrillation or asystole.

MANAGEMENT

(1) Attach an ECG monitor to the patient, gain intravenous access and give 10% calcium chloride 5–10 ml slowly i.v. for life-threatening ECG changes.

(2) Lower the serum potassium rapidly with:
- (i)   50% dextrose 50 ml i.v. with 10 U of soluble insulin;
- (ii) 8.4% sodium bicarbonate 50 ml i.v., providing there is no danger of sodium overload.

(3) Refer the patient immediately to the medical team. Urgent haemodialysis or peritoneal dialysis may be necessary, particularly in known renal failure.

THE COLLAPSED OR UNCONSCIOUS PATIENT

The aim is to resuscitate the patient, treat urgent precipitating conditions, and to build up a picture of the situation. The definitive diagnosis may not be made in the A&E department.

MANAGEMENT

(1) (i)   If the patient is unconscious, clear the airway by tilting the head and lifting the chin and remove dentures, vomit, or blood with a quick sweep round the mouth with the gloved finger.

(ii) In trauma cases open the airway with the jaw thrust only, avoiding movement of the neck.

(iii) Insert an oropharyngeal airway and give oxygen. Attach a cardiac monitor and pulse oximeter to the patient. Aim for an oxygen saturation above 94%.

(iv) If there is no gag reflex, call the anaesthetist urgently to insert an endotracheal tube.

(2) If no pulse is felt, commence cardiopulmonary resuscitation (see page 2).

(3) Otherwise:
    (i)   If there is any suggestion of face, head or neck trauma, apply a semirigid collar before moving the patient.
    (ii)   Remove all the patient's clothing.
(4) (i)   Insert an intravenous cannula and take blood for haemoglobin, blood sugar, electrolytes, LFTs, blood culture and drug screen.
    (ii)   Give 50 ml of 50% dextrose i.v., if the Glucostix is low.
         (a) Remember that dextrose can precipitate Wernicke's encephalopathy in the alcoholic or malnourished patient, who requires thiamine 100 mg i.v. immediately.
(5) Record the pulse, BP, temperature (if 35°C, repeat with a low reading thermometer to exclude hypothermia) and the pupil size and reaction.
(6) If the pupils are pinpoint, give the patient naloxone 0.8–2 mg i.v. to reverse narcotic poisoning. Consider other conditions requiring urgent action:
    (i)   *Tension pneumothorax.*
         (a) This usually follows trauma, especially if positive pressure ventilation is being given.
         (b) Insert a large-bore cannula or intercostal drain without waiting for an x-ray (see page 10).
    (ii)   *Cardiac arrhythmia.* Treat as necessary after recording a formal 12-lead ECG (see page 16).
    (iii) *Exsanguination.*
         (a) Bleeding may be obvious or concealed, coming from the gastrointestinal tract, an aortic aneurysm or a ruptured ectopic pregnancy.
         (b) Cross-match blood, give intravenous fluids and refer the patient for an urgent surgical opinion.
    (iv) *Anaphylaxis.*
         (a) This may follow drug therapy or food ingestion, a bee sting or intravenous contrast administration.

      (b) Give 0.3–0.5 ml of 1 in 1000 adrenaline intramuscularly, repeated as necessary.

      (c) If there is circulatory collapse, give 1 in 10 000 adrenaline 0.75–1.5 µg/kg i.e. 50–100 µg or 0.5–1.0 ml slowly intravenously for a 70-kg patient (see page 107).

   (v) *Extradural haemorrhage.*

      (a) This may follow even trivial trauma. Look for a local bruise on the scalp, for instance in the temporoparietal area over the middle meningeal artery territory.

      (b) Watch out for deterioration in the level of consciousness, ultimately with the development of Cheyne–Stokes breathing and a unilateral fixed, dilated pupil.

      (c) Call the anaesthetist to pass a cuffed endotracheal tube if not already in place.

      (d) Refer the patient immediately to the surgical team, before the latter signs develop. Arrange an urgent head CT scan.

(7) The most common causes of an unconscious patient are:
   (i)   poisoning (accidental or deliberate, including alcohol);
   (ii)   hypoglycaemia;
   (iii) postictal state;
   (iv) stroke;
   (v)   head injury;
   (vi) subarachnoid haemorrhage;
   (vii) respiratory failure;
   (viii) hypotension — including cardiac arrhythmia or myocardial infarction.

(8) Less common causes of an unconscious patient are:
   (i)   meningitis or encephalitis;
   (ii)   hepatic or renal failure;
   (iii) septicaemia;
   (iv) subdural haematoma;
   (v)   hyperglycaemia;
   (vi) hypothermia.

(9) Rare causes of an unconscious patient are:
   (i)   cerebral space-occupying lesion;

    (ii)   Addison's disease;

    (iii)   myxoedema;

    (iv)   hypertensive encephalopathy;

    (v)   hyponatraemia or hypercalcaemia.

(10) Finally, in those who have recently been abroad, consider:

    (i)   cerebral malaria;

    (ii)   typhus, yellow fever, trypanosomiasis and typhoid. These four lists may seem daunting, but aim to build up a picture of the events as follows.

(11) History:

    (i)   Any clues from relatives, passers-by or ambulance crew?

    (ii)   Any prior medical or surgical conditions?

    (iii)   Any known drug therapy or abuse?

    (iv)   Any witnessed fit, trauma, alcohol or drug ingestion?

    (v)   Any recent travel abroad?

(12) Further examination:

    (i)   Search the clothing for a diabetic card, steroid card or outpatient card.

    (ii)   Look particularly for signs of trauma, needle puncture marks or petechiae on the skin.

    (iii)   Reassess the vital signs including the temperature.

    (iv)   Examine the front of the chest, feel the abdomen and examine the back, inspect the perineum and perform a rectal examination.

    (v)   Reassess the neurological state, including the level of consciousness using the Glasgow Coma Scale (see page 128), the pupil responses, eye movements and fundi.

        (a)   Exclude any neck stiffness and assess the muscle power, tone and reflexes, including the plantar responses.

(13) Perform:

    (i)   CXR, ECG and arterial blood gases.

    (ii)   Lateral cervical spine x-ray and pelvic x-ray in trauma cases.

    (iii)   Head CT scan if intracranial pathology is suspected or cannot be excluded.

Having treated any urgent conditions and built up a list of the likely causes of unconsciousness, refer the patient to the medical or surgical team, if they are not already involved.

ACUTE NEUROLOGICAL CONDITIONS

The following neurological conditions frequently present to the accident and emergency department:
(1) faints;
(2) fits;
(3) status epilepticus;
(4) transient ischaemic attacks;
(5) strokes.
Headache is covered separately in the next chapter.

FAINTS

A faint is a loss of consciousness due to transient cerebral ischaemia from reduced perfusion, usually with a rapid onset associated with blurred vision, dizziness and sweating. A brief tonic–clonic fit may follow if perfusion remains impaired. Faints may be difficult to distinguish from fits or acute vertigo and so an eye-witness account is vital. Always interview ambulance crew or accompanying adults.

DIAGNOSIS

Causes include:
(1) Vasovagal — 'simple' faint, triggered by pain or emotion.
(2) Hypoglycaemia.
(3) Cardiac:
    (i)   arrhythmia, Stokes–Adams attack;
    (ii)   myocardial infarction;
    (iii)   stenotic valve lesion (especially aortic stenosis);
    (iv)   hypertrophic cardiomyopathy.
(4) Vascular:
    (i)   carotid sinus hypersensitivity;
    (ii)   pulmonary embolism.

(5) Haemorrhage:
    (i)   haematemesis;
    (ii)   melaena;
    (iii)   concealed (aortic aneurysm or ectopic pregnancy).
(6) Neurological:
    (i)   subarachnoid haemorrhage;
    (ii)   vertebrobasilar insufficiency.
(7) Cough or micturition syncope.
(8) Postural hypotension:
    (i)   diabetes, hypoadrenalism;
    (ii)   Parkinson's disease;
    (iii)   drugs:
        (a) phenothiazines;
        (b) tricyclic antidepressants;
        (c) antihypertensives, e.g. captopril, prazosin;
        (d) diuretics;
        (e) nitrates;
        (f) levodopa.

MANAGEMENT

This is aimed at excluding the more serious of the conditions above, e.g. cardiac disease or haemorrhage.

(1) Carefully examine all patients looking for hypotension (postural), a cardiac lesion, an abdominal mass or tenderness, and focal neurological signs.
(2) Check the Glucostix for hypoglycaemia, ECG and other investigations as indicated (FBC, U&E, G&S and CXR).
(3) Refer the patient to the medical or surgical team as appropriate, or for outpatient follow-up if no immediately life-threatening cause is found. A 24-hour ambulatory ECG may help, particularly in unexplained recurrent syncope.
(4) Inform the general practitioner by telephone or by letter if the patient is discharged.

FITS

DIAGNOSIS

(1) An eye-witness account is crucial to establish the diagnosis. Helpful indicators of a true epileptic seizure having occurred are:

  (i)   bitten tongue, urinary incontinence;
  (ii)   preceding aura or proceeding drowsiness;
  (iii) known epilepsy.
(2) In known epileptics the commonest causes of fits are:
  (i)   not taking their medication;
  (ii)   alcohol abuse (withdrawal or excess);
  (iii) intercurrent infection (remember meningitis);
  (iv)   head injury;
  (v)   hypoglycaemia.
(3) In nonepileptic patients presenting with a first fit or a
    sporadic fit, never diagnose new-onset epilepsy until the
    following are excluded:
  (i)   hypoglycaemia;
  (ii)   head injury;
  (iii) infection — especially meningitis and encephalitis
         (or a febrile fit in a child);
  (iv)   drug withdrawal, e.g. alcohol, benzodiazepine,
         narcotics and cocaine;
  (v)   acute poisoning, e.g. alcohol, theophylline,
         cocaine, amphetamine and tricyclics;
  (vi)   intracranial pathology:
         (a) space-occupying lesion;
         (b) cerebral ischaemia;
         (c) subarachnoid or intracerebral haemorrhage;
  (vii) hypoxia;
  (viii) hyponatraemia, hypocalcaemia, uraemia and
         eclampsia.

Note: the above acute symptomatic causes of grand mal fits must
also be excluded particularly in status epilepticus (see page 51).

MANAGEMENT

(1) Check a Glucostix and if it is low, take blood for a
    laboratory glucose estimation and give 50 ml of 50%
    dextrose i.v. (or glucagon 1 mg i.m. if venous access is
    impossible).
(2) If the patient is fitting, or the fit recurs, give diazepam
    (Diazemuls) 5–10 mg i.v. and oxygen via a face mask, to
    maintain the oxygen saturation above 94%.

(3) Do *not* attempt to wedge the mouth open; make sure the head is protected from harm and turn the patient semiprone.

(4) Proceed to FBC, U&E, LFTs, drug screen, blood culture, blood gases, CXR, ECG and CT scan as indicated clinically, and send urgent anticonvulsant levels if the patient is on treatment.

(5) Refer the following patients to the medical team:
  (i)   a first fit, or a suspected underlying cause such as meningitis, tumour, etc.;
  (ii) a fit exceeding 5 min, or recurrent fits, especially if there is no full recovery between them;
  (iii) residual focal CNS signs;
  (iv) a fit following a head injury (refer to the surgeons).

(6) A previously diagnosed epileptic may be discharged home if:
  (i)   a rapid, full recovery is made;
  (ii) the fit lasted less than 5 min and was not associated with trauma either before or during the fit;
  (iii) there are no residual focal CNS signs and the level of consciousness is normal;
  (iv) their usual medication is adequate and being taken;
  (v)   there is an adult to accompany the patient.

(7) It is important to inform the general practitioner by telephone or letter on discharging the patient, and if the patient is referred to the neurology clinic for follow-up.

STATUS EPILEPTICUS

Two or more seizures without full recovery of consciousness inbetween, or recurrent epileptic seizures for more than 30 min.

MANAGEMENT

(1) Give the patient oxygen via a face mask, attach a cardiac monitor and pulse oximeter, and aim for an oxygen saturation above 94%.

(2) Check the blood sugar:
    (i)   if it is low, give 50 ml of 50% dextrose intra-venously;
    (ii)   if chronic alcoholism or malnutrition is likely, give thiamine 100 mg i.v. in addition, to avoid precipitating Wernicke's encephalopathy.

(3) Give diazepam (Diazemuls) 5–10 mg i.v. (never i.m.), but beware causing respiratory depression, bradycardia and hypotension especially in the elderly.

(4) If the patient is still fitting, call the medical team urgently:
    (i)   Repeat the intravenous diazepam (Diazemuls);
    (ii)   Give intravenous phenytoin 15 mg/kg no faster than 50 mg/min by slow bolus or as an infusion in 250 ml normal saline over 30 min (never in dextrose).

(5) Other drugs that may be used include phenobarbitone 10–20 mg/kg i.v. no faster than 100 mg/min, 0.8% chlormethiazole or clonazepam.

(6) Occasionally, if intravenous access is impossible:
    (i)   Give rectal diazepam, especially in children, via a rectal tube (Stesolid 5 mg or 10 mg in 2.5 ml) or use parenteral diazepam solution (Valium) given through a small syringe (see page 290).
    (ii)   Give paraldehyde 0.15 ml/kg i.m. or 0.3–0.5 ml/kg rectally diluted 1:10 with normal saline or vegetable oil if fitting persists (check current prescribing information with manufacturer).

TRANSIENT ISCHAEMIC ATTACKS (TIA)

Transient ischaemic attacks are episodes of transient focal neurological deficit, lasting for less than 24 h (often less than 10 min). They may recur and are important in that they may herald a major stroke or other serious vascular event (10% per year).

DIAGNOSIS

(1) The causes may be considered in three groups.
    (i)   Embolic:

        (a) cardiac — post myocardial infarction, atrial fibrillation, mitral stenosis, valve prostheses;

        (b) extracranial vessels — carotid stenosis, narrowed vertebral artery.

    (ii) Reduced cerebral perfusion:

        (a) hypotension from hypovolaemia, drugs or a cardiac arrhythmia;

        (b) hypertension (especially in hypertensive encephalopathy);

        (c) polycythaemia, paraproteinaemia, antiphospholipid antibodies;

        (d) vasculitis, e.g. temporal arteritis, systemic lupus erythematosus, polyarteritis nodosa or syphilis.

    (iii) Lack of nutrients:

        (a) anaemia;

        (b) hypoglycaemia.

(2) They present clinically as:

    (i) Carotid territory dysfunction causing hemiparesis, hemianaesthesia, hemianopia, dysphasia, dysarthria and amaurosis fugax (transitory monocular blindness).

    (ii) Vertebrobasilar territory dysfunction causing combinations of tetraparesis, crossed sensory symptoms, diplopia, nystagmus, ataxia, vertigo and cortical blindness.

(3) Examination must therefore include:

    (i) Checking the heart sounds, blood pressure (in both arms), listening for carotid bruits and a full neurological assessment.

    (ii) Checking the blood sugar, FBC, ESR, coagulation profile, U&E, LFTs, CXR and ECG.

MANAGEMENT

(1) Refer the patient to the medical team if:

    (i) an embolic source is suspected;

    (ii) carotid stenosis is suspected;

    (iii) the patient is hypertensive with a diastolic blood pressure over 110 mmHg;

    (iv)   a significant systemic disorder is suspected;
    (v)   TIA are recurring over a period of hours or are of progressive severity and intensity;
    (vi)   a severe transient neurological deficit occurred or there are residual neurological findings.

(2) A CT scan will distinguish intracranial haemorrhage and doppler carotid ultrasound significant carotid stenosis. Arrange these in consultation with the medical team.

(3) Otherwise, if complete recovery has occurred, consider starting a beta blocker or diuretic for mild hypertension and refer to medical outpatients.

(4) In the remainder of cases, commence low-dose aspirin 75 mg once daily and refer to medical outpatients or to the general practitioner.

Note: remember that patients can present with the consequences of their TIA, e.g. a head injury, Colles' fracture, or fracture of the neck of femur.

STROKES

These are due to a vascular disturbance producing a focal neurological deficit for over 24 h.

DIAGNOSIS

(1) The causes include:
    (i)   Cerebral infarction (80%):
        (a) cerebral thrombosis from atherosclerosis, hypertension or rarely arteritis, etc;
        (b) cerebral embolism from atrial fibrillation, mitral stenosis, postmyocardial infarction or from atheromatous plaques in a neck vessel.
    (ii)   Cerebral haemorrhage (20%):
        (a) intracerebral haemorrhage associated with hypertension or rarely intracranial tumour and bleeding disorders including anticoagulation;
        (b) subarachnoid haemorrhage from ruptured berry aneurysm or arteriovenous malformation.

(2) Presentation may give a clue to aetiology:

    (i)   Cerebral thrombosis is often preceded by a TIA and the neurological deficit usually progresses gradually. Headache and loss of consciousness are uncommon.

    (ii)   Cerebral embolism causes a sudden, complete neurological deficit.

    (iii)   Intracerebral haemorrhage causes sudden onset of headache, vomiting, stupor or coma with a rapidly progressive neurological deficit.

    (iv)   Subarachnoid haemorrhage is heralded by:

        (a)   sudden severe headache often after exertion, associated with meningism i.e. stiff neck, photophobia, vomiting and Kernig's sign (see page 57).

        (b)   confusion or lethargy which are common, or focal neurological deficit and coma which are rare and serious.

(3) Record the vital signs including the temperature, pulse, blood pressure and respiratory rate.

(4) Perform a careful neurological examination recording the progression of symptoms and signs.

MANAGEMENT

This is essentially supportive.

(1) If the patient is unconscious:

    (i)   Open the airway by tilting the head and lifting the chin, insert an oropharyngeal airway and give oxygen;

    (ii)   Place the patient in the left lateral position. Call an anaesthetist urgently to pass a cuffed endotracheal tube if the gag reflex is absent.

(2) Otherwise, commence oxygen, attach a cardiac monitor and pulse oximeter to the patient. Aim for an oxygen saturation above 94%.

(3) Gain intravenous access and send blood for FBC, ESR, coagulation profile, U&E, LFTs and blood sugar. Give 50 ml of 50% dextrose i.v. if the Glucostix is low. Catheterise the bladder.

(4) Obtain an ECG, CXR and arrange an urgent CT head scan.

(5) Refer the patient to the medical team for admission and definitive diagnosis.

    (i)   Avoid the temptation to treat raised blood pressure acutely unless hypertensive encephalopathy (see page 59) or aortic dissection (see page 19) are suspected.

    (ii)   A cerebellar stroke presenting with headache, dizziness, vertigo, truncal or limb ataxia and gaze palsy may be amenable to urgent neurosurgical intervention.

HEADACHE

DIFFERENTIAL DIAGNOSIS

Consider the serious or life-threatening diagnoses first:
(1) meningitis;
(2) subarachnoid haemorrhage;
(3) space-occupying lesion;
(4) hypertensive encephalopathy;
(5) temporal arteritis.

The majority however will be due to:
(6) migraine;
(7) tension headache;
(8) post-traumatic headache;
(9) disease in other cranial structures.

The history is vital as physical signs may be lacking even in the serious group. A new headache or a change in quality of a usual one must be evaluated carefully.

MENINGITIS

DIAGNOSIS

(1) Prodromal malaise, followed by generalised headache, fever, vomiting and drowsiness occur progressing to confusion or coma.

(2) A pyrexia, photophobia and neck stiffness are found. Localised cranial nerve palsies or fits may occur.

(3) Kernig's sign of meningeal irritation elicits pain and spasm in the hamstrings on attempted knee extension with the hip flexed.

(4) A petechial rash suggests meningococcal septicaemia.

MANAGEMENT

(1) Give the patient oxygen and gain intravenous access. Send blood for FBC, U&E, blood sugar, viral studies and blood culture.

(2) Commence a normal saline infusion and perform a CXR.

(3) Refer the patient immediately to the medical team:

    (i)   A CT scan should precede a lumbar puncture if there are focal neurological signs or papilloedema.

    (ii)   Neither should delay the prompt start of intravenous antibiotics, which should be given as soon as the diagnosis is suspected:

        (a) Give benzylpenicillin 3 Mu (1.8 g) i.v. and ceftriaxone 2 g i.v.

SUBARACHNOID HAEMORRHAGE

DIAGNOSIS

(1) Hypertension, polycystic kidneys and coarctation of the aorta are associated with berry aneurysm whose rupture causes the majority of cases.

(2) Prodromal episodes of headache or diplopia due to 'warning leaks' may precede a sudden, severe headache often following exertion.

(3) Lethargy, nausea, vomiting and meningism with photophobia and neck stiffness occur, although fever is usually absent. A III nerve oculomotor palsy suggests bleeding from a posterior communicating artery aneurysm.

(4) Presentation may be with acute confusion, transient loss of consciousness or coma, when a stiff neck and subhyaloid (preretinal) haemorrhages are useful diagnostic pointers.

MANAGEMENT

(1) Give the patient oxygen and nurse head upwards. Aim for an oxygen saturation above 94%.

(2) Gain intravenous access and send blood for FBC, U&E, blood sugar and perform an ECG and CXR.

(3) Give diazepam (Diazemuls) 5 mg i.v. for fits or severe agitation. Give dihydrocodeine 30–60 mg orally or occasionally morphine 2.5–5 mg i.v. for pain relief, with an antiemetic such as metoclopramide 10 mg i.v.

(4) Refer the patient to the medical team or neurosurgical unit:

    (i) Arrange a CT scan urgently to confirm the diagnosis.

    (ii) Perform a lumbar puncture if the CT scan is negative or unavailable, providing there are no focal neurological signs or papilloedema.

        (a) Always request xanthochromia studies by spectrophotometry of the CSF to differentiate a traumatic tap (absent), from a true subarachnoid haemorrhage (positive).

    (iii) Consider a nimodipine infusion at 1 mg/h, increased to 2 mg/h after 2 h if the blood pressure is stable, or nimodipine 60 mg orally 4-hourly when the diagnosis is confirmed.

SPACE-OCCUPYING LESION

DIAGNOSIS

(1) Causes include an intracranial haematoma, cerebral tumour or cerebral abscess.

(2) The headaches become progressively more frequent and severe, worse in the mornings and exacerbated by coughing, bending or straining.

(3) Vomiting without nausea occurs and focal neurological signs develop ranging from subtle personality changes, ataxia, visual problems to cranial nerve palsies, hemiparesis and seizures.

(4) Papilloedema is seen with loss of venous pulsation and blurring of the disc margin with filling in of the optic cup as the earliest signs on fundoscopy.

MANAGEMENT

(1) Give oxygen and treat seizures with diazepam (Diazemuls) 5 mg i.v.
(2) Perform a CXR to look for a primary tumour and arrange a CT head scan. If this is not immediately available, consider a skull x-ray to look for a fracture, shift of the pineal, bony erosion or sclerosis and eroded posterior clinoids or pituitary fossa floor.
(3) Refer any patient with a possible extradural or subdural to the neurosurgical team.
(4) Otherwise refer the patient to the medical team for full investigation.

HYPERTENSIVE ENCEPHALOPATHY

DIAGNOSIS

(1) An acute hypertensive crisis causing severe hypertension (diastolic over 140 mmHg), headache, confusion, vomiting, deteriorating vision, and retinal haemorrhages, exudates or papilloedema.
(2) Focal neurological signs, fits and coma develop later.

MANAGEMENT

(1) Give the patient oxygen, attach a cardiac monitor and pulse oximeter and aim for an oxygen saturation above 94%.
(2) Gain intravenous access and send blood for FBC, U&E, LFTs and blood sugar.
(3) Request a CXR and perform an ECG.
(4) Treat the blood pressure immediately with nifedipine 10 mg orally or sublingually repeated as necessary to achieve a diastolic pressure of 100–110 mmHg.
(5) Refer the patient to the medical team for blood pressure control and to observe for the complications of heart failure, aortic dissection, intracranial haemorrhage and renal impairment.

TEMPORAL ARTERITIS

DIAGNOSIS

(1) Severe, bitemporal headache often associated with a history of malaise, weight loss and myalgia occurring in a patient over 50 years old is typical.

(2) Localised scalp tenderness, hyperaesthesia and decreased temporal arterial pulsation are seen, occasionally with pain on chewing (jaw claudication).

(3) The immediate danger is sudden visual loss due to ophthalmic artery involvement which may affect both eyes if treatment is delayed.

MANAGEMENT

(1) Send blood for an urgent ESR.

(2) Commence prednisolone 60 mg orally.

(3) Refer the patient to the medical or ophthalmology team for admission for temporal artery biopsy and high-dose steroid therapy.

MIGRAINE

DIAGNOSIS

(1) Classic migraine attacks begin before the age of 40 years with a positive family history in up to 70%.

   (i)   A visual prodrome with flashing lights, fortification spectra, teichopsia (zigzag lines of light) and a central scotoma is usual (i.e. migraine with aura).

   (ii)   Hemianopia, hemisensory, dysphasic or hemiplegic aura is less common.

   (iii) Headache is unilateral, throbbing or pulsating, recurrent and periodic lasting 4 h to 3 days.

   (iv) Nausea, vomiting, photophobia and phonophobia are associated.

(2) Common migraine is more usual in females and resembles classic migraine though may be bilateral and lacks the typical prodrome (i.e. migraine without aura).

(3) Rare variants include hemiplegic, ophthalmoplegic and vertebrobasilar migraine.

MANAGEMENT

(1) Nurse the patient in a darkened room, give oxygen by face mask and an analgesic such as paracetamol 500 mg and codeine phosphate 8 mg (co-codamol) two tablets orally.
(2) Give an antiemetic such as metoclopramide (Maxolon) 10 mg i.v. or prochlorperazine (Stemetil) 12.5 mg i.m. for vomiting.
(3) Give sumatriptan 6 mg s.c. only for resistant headache:
   (i)   Side effects of tingling, heat and flushing may occur or rarely chest pain and tightness.
   (ii) Sumatriptan is thus contra-indicated in known coronary artery disease, previous myocardial infarction and in patients with possible unrecognised coronary artery disease, e.g. post-menopausal women or men over 40 with risk factors.
   (iii) It is also contra-indicated within 24 h of ergotamine-containing therapy.
(4) Discharge the patient back to the general practitioner having discussed precipitating factors such as chocolate, cheese, alcohol, hunger, etc. that could be avoided.

TENSION HEADACHE

DIAGNOSIS

(1) Women are more commonly affected with headaches associated with stress but lacking any prodrome.
(2) The pain comes on gradually and is bilateral, dull, constant and band-like.
(3) Mild nausea, phonophobia and photophobia can occur though vomiting is rare. Headaches often become chronic.

MANAGEMENT

(1) Give the patient an analgesic such as paracetamol 500 mg and codeine phosphate 8 mg (co-codamol) two tablets orally.
(2) Reassure the patient and discharge back to the care of the general practitioner.

POST-TRAUMATIC HEADACHE

DIAGNOSIS

(1) Headache following head injury may begin immediately or after a few days and is present in up to 30% of patients at 6 weeks after mild concussion.
(2) Inability to concentrate, dizziness, insomnia, irritability even depression may develop, known as the 'post-concussion syndrome'.

MANAGEMENT

(1) Persistent worsening of headache, clouding of consciousness or focal neurological signs require urgent CT scan and referral to the neurosurgical team to exclude a subdural haematoma.
(2) Otherwise treatment is supportive including analgesics, rest and reassurance that complete recovery is the rule.
(3) Refer the patient back to the general practitioner, as symptoms may persist for up to 1 year.

DISEASE IN OTHER CRANIAL STRUCTURES

DIAGNOSIS AND MANAGEMENT

(1) Glaucoma (see page 326), iritis (see page 325), otitis media (see page 300), sinusitis or dental caries may all present with headache.
(2) Treatment is aimed at the underlying condition.

ACUTE POISONING

Most cases will be acts of deliberate self-harm in the adult, whereas in children they are usually accidental.

Initially, all cases are managed as medical emergencies, including resuscitation, substance identification and elimination, specific and nonspecific treatment and a period of observation.

Thereafter, cases may require psychiatric assessment. Remember that an apparently trivial act of self-harm may still indicate serious suicidal intent (see page 362).

DIAGNOSIS

(1) Consider acute poisoning in any unconscious patient or patient exhibiting bizarre behaviour, or in unexplained metabolic, respiratory and cardiovascular problems.

(2) Obtain information from any witnesses to the circumstances of the poisoning, ask if tablets were found and the approximate time of their ingestion.

(3) Corroborate the history with the patient, although he or she may be unable to remember exactly what was taken and when, or may deliberately mislead.

(4) Remember that two or more drugs are taken in 30% of cases and alcohol is a common adjunct.

MANAGEMENT

This will depend if the patient is unconscious or conscious:

(1) If the patient is unconscious or collapsed:

(i) Clear the airway by extending the head, remove dentures, vomit or blood by a quick sweep round the mouth with a gloved finger, insert an oropharyngeal airway and give oxygen via a face mask.

(ii) If the patient is not breathing or the gag reflex is absent, insert an oropharyngeal (Guedel) airway and use an Ambu or Laerdal bag and face mask to ventilate the patient. Call the anaesthetist urgently to pass a cuffed endotracheal tube.

(iii) Record the pulse, blood pressure, respiratory rate and temperature (beware of hypothermia) and attach a cardiac monitor and pulse oximeter to the patient. Aim for an oxygen saturation above 94%.

(iv) Gain venous access. Take blood for glucose, U&E and a drug screen and give:

    (a) 50 ml of 50% dextrose i.v. if the Glucostix is low;

    (b) naloxone 0.8–2 mg i.v. if the pupils are pinpoint.

(v) Maintain the circulation with an infusion of normal saline unless the hypotension is secondary to an arrhythmia or myocardial depression, when specific drug therapy and inotropic support with dopamine or dobutamine are indicated (see page 12).

(vi) Check the arterial blood gases, CXR and ECG:

    (a) metabolic acidosis occurs with salicylate, methanol, ethanol, iron and ethylene glycol poisoning.

(vii) If the patient is cardiovascularly stable and the airway is protected by a cuffed endotracheal tube, perform gastric lavage:

    (a) This must not be done if there is known ingestion of a corrosive substance, oil or petrol, or it is suspected from scalding of the lips and mouth or a characteristic foetor.

    (b) Save a 20-ml sample of the aspirate for a drug screen.

    (c) Pass activated charcoal 50 g in 100–200 ml water plus 70% sorbitol 50 ml as a cathartic down the lavage tube prior to removal (see page 66). Do not add the sorbitol if there is diarrhoea, intestinal obstruction or an ileus.

(viii) Refer the patient urgently to the medical team, if they are not already involved.

(2) If the patient is conscious, do not be misled as serious poisoning may still have occurred and the effects may be delayed.

(i) Obtain a history of the substances taken, the time of ingestion, associated alcohol consumption, current medical conditions and any toxic effects experienced from the poisoning.

(ii) Examine for clues to the substance taken:
- (a) dilated pupils — tricyclics, amphetamine, cocaine, antihistamines, anticholinergics;
- (b) pinpoint pupils — opiates (remember Lomotil), organophosphates;
- (c) nystagmus — alcohol, benzodiazepines, phenytoin;
- (d) nasal bleeding or perioral sores — solvent abuse;
- (e) hyperventilation — salicylate.

(iii) Check the vital signs and examine the chest for signs of aspiration.

(iv) Send blood routinely for a paracetamol level.
- (a) This drug may have been taken and the patient seriously poisoned with no overt signs initially. Ask the laboratory staff also to save a sample of serum.
- (b) Other drug levels are only indicated in specific cases according to the history and physical findings.
- (c) Send additional blood for U&E, blood sugar and osmolarity as appropriate and consider requesting an ECG and CXR.

(v) Gastric lavage:
- (a) Perform gastric lavage in the occasional patient who presents early within 1–2 hours of ingestion and shows serious clinical features of toxicity or has taken a potentially lethal amount of drug. It should no longer be routine in mild to moderate poisoning.
- (b) Position the patient head down in the left lateral position and use 200–300 ml of warm tap water for each lavage cycle.
- (c) If the patient has a reduced cough or gag reflex, the airway *must* first be protected by a cuffed endotracheal tube.

(d) Corrosive, caustic or petroleum-derivative ingestion are absolute contraindications to lavage.

(e) Pass activated charcoal 50 g down the lavage tube before removal (see below).

(f) Syrup of ipecacuanha is preferred in children unless unconscious and seriously poisoned, when gastric lavage (with the airway protected) is indicated.

(vi) Induced emesis:

(a) If a patient refuses gastric lavage, or in conscious children as a preferred alternative, use syrup of ipecacuanha 15 ml for a child and 30 ml for an adult, followed by 200 ml of water to cause emesis.

(b) Repeat this after 30 min if there is no response, providing the patient is still fully conscious.

(c) Never use ipecacuanha if it is known that corrosive material, oil or petrol were ingested or if the substance taken could induce seizures or drowsiness before the emesis has occurred, as the patient may then aspirate vomitus.

(vii) Activated charcoal:

(a) This is gaining favour as the first-line measure to reduce the absorption of many drugs, ideally administered within 4 h of their ingestion.

(b) The dose is 50 g for adults (or 1 g/kg body weight in children) in 100–200 ml water with 70% sorbitol 50 ml as a slurry given orally or down the lavage tube.

(c) Do not add the sorbitol if the patient has severe diarrhoea, intestinal obstruction or an ileus.

(d) Give repeated 25 g doses without sorbitol every 4 h in salicylate, theophylline, digoxin, carbamazepine, quinine, phenytoin and phenobarbitone poisoning.

(e) Warn the patient charcoal is somewhat unpalatable and will turn the stools black.

(f) Avoid if an oral antidote or syrup of ipecacuanha is to be given.

(g) Remember also that it is not effective for poisoning by cyanide, alcohols, iron, lithium, acid, alkali, petroleum or pesticides.

(viii) Refer the patient to the medical team or admit to the observation ward, once relevant drug levels are known and the clinical severity of the poisoning is apparent.

SPECIFIC POISONS

Advice on the management of all types of poisoning may be obtained from the following Poisons Information Centres:

London
  National Poisons Information Service   0171 635 9191
Birmingham
  West Midlands Poisons Unit   0121 554 3801
Leeds
  Leeds Poisons Information Service   0113 243 0715
Newcastle
  Northern Regional Drug and   0191 232 5131
  Therapeutics Centre
Edinburgh
  Scottish Poisons Information Bureau   0131 229 2477
Cardiff
  Welsh National Poisons Unit   01222 709901
Belfast
  Northern Ireland Drugs and Poisons
  Information Service   01232 240503
Dublin
  Poisons Information Centre   0001 379966

SALICYLATES

DIAGNOSIS

(1) The patient is restless, flushed, sweating, hyperventilating, and may complain of nausea, vomiting, tinnitus or deafness.

(2) Confusion, coma, fits, or cardiac arrest are rare and signify severe poisoning.

(3) Complicated metabolic effects occur including:
- (i)   hypokalaemic alkalosis (vomiting);
- (ii) respiratory alkalosis (hyperventilation);
- (iii) metabolic acidosis (several causes);
- (iv) dehydration and hyperpyrexia;
- (v)   hypoglycaemia or hyperglycaemia;
- (vi) bleeding tendency (low prothrombin and platelet effect);
- (vii) pulmonary oedema (hypersensitivity).

MANAGEMENT

(1) Give activated charcoal 50 g, or perform gastric lavage followed by activated charcoal 50 g, for recent serious poisoning.

(2) Check levels early. In adults symptoms occur at 2.2 mmol/l and toxicity is serious over 3.3 mmol/l. Repeat the level at least once to monitor for further drug absorption.

(3) Check FBC, U&E, blood sugar, PTI and blood gases if the salicylate level is high, rising or the patient is symptomatic.

(4) Commence intravenous normal saline and refer all serious cases with levels over 3.3 mmol/l or markedly symptomatic to the medical team. Otherwise observe in the overnight ward.

(5) Haemodialysis may be considered for severe poisoning or a level over 5.1 mmol/l.

PARACETAMOL

DIAGNOSIS

(1) The initial symptom may be nausea alone, but the danger is delayed fulminant hepatic failure causing abdominal pain, vomiting, hypoglycaemia, tender hepatomegaly, jaundice, encephalopathy and death.

(2) Patients who regularly take enzyme-inducing drugs such

as phenytoin, carbamazepine, phenobarbitone and rifampicin or alcohol are at increased risk of hepatotoxicity. Starvation and debilitating illness such as AIDS may also increase the risk.

(3) A potentially fatal paracetamol dose is 12 g, although in patients on enzyme-inducing drugs it may be as low as 7.5 g (15 tablets).

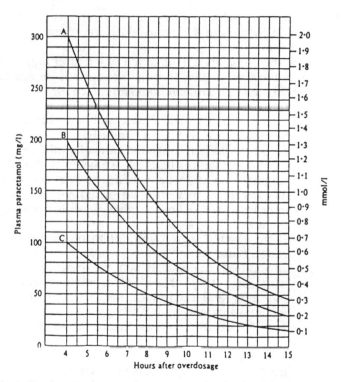

Fig. 4. Treatment nomogram for paracetamol poisoning. Line B: specific treatment is indicated above this line. Line C: specific treatment is indicated above this line in patients who regularly take enzyme–inducing drugs such as phenytoin, carbamazepine, phenobarbitone and rifampicin or alcohol. Line A: 90% of untreated patients will develop ALT (alanine transaminase) levels over 1000 IU/l and most fatal cases will be above this line.
(Reproduced with permission from Proudfoot A.T. (1993). *Acute Poisoning Diagnosis and Management*, 2nd edn. Oxford: Butterworth–Heinemann.)

(4) N-acetylcysteine (Parvolex) is a highly effective antidote provided it is commenced within 8 h of poisoning.

    (i)   Figure 4 is a treatment nomogram indicating when to use N-acetylcysteine.

MANAGEMENT

(1) Give activated charcoal 50 g, or perform gastric lavage followed by activated charcoal 50 g, for recent serious poisoning.

(2) Check the blood level a minimum of 4 h after ingestion and determine if the specific antidote is indicated according to the treatment nomogram (see Fig. 4).

(3) Commence N-acetylcysteine i.v. immediately if the blood level is in the toxic range, and send blood for baseline blood sugar, U&E, PTI and LFTs.

    (i)   However, if the result of the paracetamol level will not be available within an estimated 8 h of the original ingestion, commence N-acetylcysteine anyway in a patient with a potentially fatal overdose (see definition above) whilst awaiting the level.

    (ii)   If the level is then found not to be in the toxic range, cease the infusion.

    (iii)   In addition, give N-acetylcysteine to every patient who presents 15 h or longer after significant poisoning and send blood for serum creatinine, PTI and a paracetamol level:

        (a)   Discuss the further management of these patients presenting late with a Poisons Information Centre.

(4) Give intravenous N-acetylcysteine (Parvolex) 150 mg/kg in 200 ml 5% dextrose over 15 min, followed by 50 mg/kg in 500 ml 5% dextrose over 4 h, then 100 mg/kg in 1000 ml 5% dextrose over 16 h.

    (i)   Side effects include flushing, urticaria, wheeze and hypotension:

        (a)   Stop the infusion and give chlorpheniramine 10 mg i.v. and hydrocortisone 200 mg i.v.;

(b) Once the adverse effects have settled, restart the N-acetylcysteine infusion cautiously at the lowest rate e.g. 100 mg/kg over 16 h.

TRICYCLIC ANTIDEPRESSANTS

DIAGNOSIS

These cause drowsiness, dilated pupils, dry mouth, tachycardia, urinary retention, progressing to fits, coma, respiratory depression, hypotension, cardiac arrhythmias and cardiac arrest.

MANAGEMENT

(1) Give activated charcoal 50 g, or perform gastric lavage, providing the airway is protected by endotracheal intubation, followed by activated charcoal 50 g in seriously poisoned patients.
(2) Perform a 12-lead ECG looking for a prolonged PR or QT interval, QRS widening or any arrhythmia:
  (i)   Give 8.4% sodium bicarbonate 1–2 ml/kg (1–2 mmol/kg) providing respirations are adequate, which may dramatically improve cardiac arrhythmias even in the absence of acidosis.
  (ii) Avoid giving an antiarrhythmic drug if possible.
(3) Call the anaesthetist to intubate the patient if the gag reflex is reduced, respirations are inadequate, convulsions occur or there are cardiac arrhythmias. Hyperventilation also improves cardiac arrhythmias, similarly to sodium bicarbonate.
(4) Refer all cases to the medical team who may arrange ECG monitoring in CCU or ITU.

BENZODIAZEPINES

DIAGNOSIS

(1) These are comparatively safe taken alone causing drowsiness, ataxia, dysarthria and nystagmus.

(2) Coma is unusual unless combined with other sedatives, alcohol or in the elderly.

MANAGEMENT

(1) Gastric lavage and activated charcoal are rarely necessary unless the patient is unconscious, when airway protection with endotracheal intubation is required first.

(2) Otherwise, give oxygen and place in the left lateral position to prevent aspiration.

(3) Flumazenil, a specific benzodiazepine antagonist, may avoid the need for intubation in severe cases and clarify the extent of benzodiazepine involvement in coma of unknown aetiology. It is rarely if ever indicated:

    (i)   Perform an ECG first to exclude additional tricyclic antidepressant poisoning suggested by:
        (a)   rate over 100 beats/min;
        (b)   QRS width over 0.1 s;
        (c)   corrected QT interval over 0.42 s.

    (ii)   If the ECG is abnormal as above suggesting tricyclic poisoning or if the patient is epileptic on long-term benzodiazepines, flumazenil must not be used.

    (iii)   Otherwise, give flumazenil 200 µg over 15 s followed by 100 µg/min up to 1 mg total.

(4) Refer all patients to the medical team for admission, particularly if flumazenil was used as there is a risk of deterioration as the flumazenil wears off.

OPIATES

DIAGNOSIS

Opiates cause respiratory depression, pinpoint pupils and hypotension. Vomiting, convulsions and pulmonary oedema may also occur.

MANAGEMENT

(1) Give naloxone 0.8–2 mg i.v. repeated at intervals of 2–3 min to a maximum of 10 mg. This has a short half-life and further doses or an infusion may be required.

(2) Therefore, refer all patients to the medical team, as they may relapse as the naloxone wears off.

Note: naloxone may be given intramuscularly or through the endotracheal tube, if venous access is difficult. Remember also to give naloxone in Lomotil and co-proxamol overdoses, and in any case of coma or respiratory depression with pinpoint pupils.

IRON

DIAGNOSIS

(1) Iron tablets are often mistaken for sweets by children.
(2) They cause haemorrhagic gastroenteritis with vomiting, bloody diarrhoea, encephalopathy, acute hepatic necrosis and hypotension.
(3) A plain abdominal x-ray may show residual whole tablets or a concretion.

MANAGEMENT

(1) Perform gastric lavage providing the airway is protected, or whole bowel lavage if there are significant numbers of tablets beyond the pylorus.
(2) Give desferrioxamine 2 g i.m. for potentially serious poisoning (greater than 60 mg elemental iron/kg body weight ingested) whilst awaiting an iron level.
(3) Send blood for haemoglobin, U&E, G&S and an iron level. An iron level in the adult of over 50 μmol/l is significant and over 90 μmol/l is serious.
(4) Refer all cases to the medical team. Admission to intensive care and intravenous desferrioxamine are required for severe cases.

DIGOXIN

DIAGNOSIS

(1) Toxicity occurs from acute overdose or in long-term therapy particularly in the elderly, associated with

hypokalaemia, renal impairment, hypercalcaemia and drugs such as quinidine and amiodarone which increase plasma digoxin concentration.
(2) Foxglove and oleander ingestion will also cause acute cardiac glycoside poisoning.
(3) Fatigue, anorexia, nausea, vomiting, diarrhoea, altered colour vision and delirium occur.
(4) Any cardiac arrhythmia may be seen, although brady-cardia, heart block, paroxysmal atrial tachycardia with block, ventricular ectopics and ventricular tachycardia are characteristic.

MANAGEMENT

(1) Give activated charcoal 50 g or perform gastric lavage followed by activated charcoal 50 g, for recent serious poisoning.
(2) Monitor the ECG and give oxygen.
(3) Send blood for U&E and a digoxin level. Toxicity occurs with levels over 2 ng/ml, although the level should be repeated after 4 h in acute poisoning.
(4) In chronic toxicity correct hypokalaemia with 20 mmol potassium i.v. per hour (1.5 g KCl), but note that in severe acute poisoning hyperkalaemia may occur.
(5) Refer the patient to the medical team for ECG monitoring. Digoxin-specific antibody fragments (Digibind) are indicated for haemodynamically unstable arrhythmias or hyperkalaemia i.e. serum potassium over 5 mmol/l in severe acute poisoning.

LITHIUM

DIAGNOSIS

(1) Lithium causes polyuria, thirst, tremor, fasciculations, slurred speech and ataxia, progressing to fits and coma.
(2) Toxicity may be inadvertently precipitated by dehydration or the use of diuretics or nonsteroidal anti-inflammatory drugs, as the therapeutic range of lithium (0.7–1.3 mmol/l) and toxic range (1.5 mmol/l or over) are close.

MANAGEMENT

(1) Check the lithium level, U&E and blood sugar.
(2) Perform gastric lavage for recent, serious poisoning but do not give activated charcoal (ineffective).
(3) Commence intravenous normal saline, or 5% dextrose if there is hypernatraemia.
(4) Refer all cases to the medical team. The patient may require peritoneal or haemodialysis if the level is over 3.5 mmol/l.

THEOPHYLLINE

DIAGNOSIS

(1) Nausea, intractable vomiting, abdominal pain, agitation, hyperventilation and tachycardia occur progressing to gastrointestinal bleeding, convulsions, coma and cardiac arrhythmias.
(2) Severe hypokalaemia and hyperglycaemia are seen.
(3) Delayed toxicity occurs with sustained-release preparations.

MANAGEMENT

(1) Give activated charcoal, or perform gastric lavage followed by activated charcoal 50 g, in recent serious poisoning.
(2) Give high-dose metoclopramide 10–40 mg i.v. for intractable vomiting.
(3) Monitor the ECG and send blood for U&E, blood sugar, arterial blood gases and theophylline level.
  (i) Toxic symptoms occur with theophylline levels over 25 mg/l.
  (ii) In acute poisoning levels over 40 mg/l are dangerous and over 60 mg/l potentially fatal.
  (iii) In chronic toxicity, levels over 20 mg/l cause symptoms and over 40 mg/l are life-threatening.
(4) Give diazepam (Diazemuls) 5–10 mg i.v. for convulsions, although endotracheal intubation may then be required.

(5) Correct fluid depletion and hypokalaemia with normal saline and potassium under ECG control.

(6) In nonasthmatic patients, hypokalaemia, hyperglycaemia and tachycardia respond to propranolol 1 mg i.v. over 1 min repeated up to a maximum of 10 mg.

(7) Refer all patients to the medical team for ECG monitoring, intensive care and possibly charcoal haemoperfusion.

BETA BLOCKERS

DIAGNOSIS

Beta blockers may cause bradycardia, hypotension, coma, convulsions and cardiogenic shock.

MANAGEMENT

(1) Give oxygen and check U&E and blood sugar.

(2) Give atropine 0.6–1.2 mg i.v. for bradycardia, up to a maximum of 0.04 mg/kg.

(3) Give activated charcoal 50 g or perform gastric lavage followed by activated charcoal 50 g, in recent serious poisoning.

(4) Refer the patient to the medical team for admission to the coronary care unit. The patient may require intravenous glucagon 50–150 µg/kg followed by an infusion, an isoprenaline infusion, or a cardiac pacemaker.

CARBON MONOXIDE

DIAGNOSIS

(1) Carbon monoxide poisoning is usually caused by a car exhaust or the combustion of fuel with an inadequate flue, e.g. a blocked domestic heater.

(2) It causes impaired consciousness, vomiting, headache, neurological signs, hypotension and arrhythmias.

(3) It should be suspected if there are several members of one household who present in a similar fashion.

MANAGEMENT

(1) Give 100% oxygen by tight-fitting mask with reservoir bag and monitor the ECG.
   (i) Remember a pulse oximeter will record a misleadingly normal oxygen saturation.
   (ii) Likewise the partial pressure of oxygen and calculated oxygen saturation will be normal on arterial blood gases. However, there may be a metabolic acidosis due to tissue hypoxia.
(2) Check the carboxyhaemoglobin level and blood gases:
   (i) A carboxyhaemoglobin level up to 9% is seen in smokers. Higher than this indicates toxic exposure, although there is no absolute correlation between the initial level and eventual outcome.
   (ii) A carboxyhaemoglobin level over 60% is likely to be associated with severe poisoning and the risk of death.
(3) Refer the patient to the medical team for treatment with mannitol for cerebral oedema, acid–base correction and general supportive measures.
(4) If the patient was found unconscious or has neurological symptoms other than headache, cardiac complications, a carboxyhaemoglobin level of 40% or is pregnant and facilities are available locally, refer to a hyperbaric oxygen unit.
   (i) The best results are achieved if hyperbaric treatment is started within 2 h of the patient being found. The Poisons Information Centres have details of local hyperbaric units.

ORGANOPHOSPHATES

DIAGNOSIS

These are widely available as insecticides.
(1) Absorption is through the skin, bronchi or orally.
(2) Weakness, agitation, headache, sweating, pinpoint pupils, salivation, lacrimation, bronchospasm, bronchorrhoea, abdominal pain and diarrhoea occur.

(3) Muscle paralysis, bradycardia, coma, convulsions and asystole occur in severe cases.

MANAGEMENT

(1) Remove soiled clothing and wash the skin wearing gloves, give oxygen and call the anaesthetist to pass an endotracheal tube for respiratory failure and severe bronchorrhoea.
(2) Perform gastric lavage for oral poisoning.
(3) Monitor the ECG and give atropine 2 mg i.v. repeated until the skin becomes dry, and pupillary dilatation and tachycardia occur.
(4) Refer the patient to the medical team. Pralidoxime 1–2 g i.v. over 10 min is indicated in severe cases presenting within 12–24 h with normal renal function.
  (i)   Pralidoxime should not be used for carbamate insecticide poisoning.

PARAQUAT

DIAGNOSIS

(1) As little as 10–15 ml of liquid paraquat (Gramoxone) is fatal.
(2) It causes oral and pharyngeal ulceration, nausea, vomiting and diarrhoea, myocarditis, hepatic and renal damage and life-threatening pulmonary oedema or progressive pulmonary fibrosis.

MANAGEMENT

(1) Gastric lavage must be performed (a rare exception to the rule concerning corrosive materials).
(2) Instil up to 1000 ml of 15% aqueous suspension of Fuller's earth into the stomach via the gastric lavage tube, and give 20% mannitol 200 ml as a cathartic. Use activated charcoal 50–100 g if Fuller's earth is unavailable.
(3) Check the blood gases but do not give oxygen initially, as this enhances the pulmonary toxicity.

(4) Refer the patient immediately to the medical team for admission to ITU.

CHLOROQUINE

DIAGNOSIS

(1) This causes nausea, vomiting, drowsiness, followed by dyspnoea, convulsions and coma.
(2) Cardiac effects include hypotension, QRS prolongation and ventricular arrhythmias.
(3) As little as 2.5–5 g may be rapidly fatal.

MANAGEMENT

(1) Give activated charcoal 50 g, or perform gastric lavage followed by activated charcoal, for recent serious poisoning.
(2) Check the U&E, and arterial blood gases and monitor the ECG.
(3) Give high-dose diazepam 1–2 mg/kg i.v. for severe cardiotoxicity, having called the anaesthetist to intubate the patient first. Inotropic support with adrenaline will also be necessary.
(4) Refer the patient to the medical team.

CYANIDE

See under smoke inhalation, page 169.

ENVIRONMENTAL EMERGENCIES

Heat illness, hypothermia and near drowning are considered together here and sports diving accidents on pages 84–7.

HEAT ILLNESS

This is predisposed to by hot weather, exercise, obesity, lack of physical fitness or acclimatisation, fever and recent alcohol intake or anticholinergic drug use.

DIAGNOSIS

(1) Mild to moderate heat illness with intact thermoregulatory mechanisms:
  - (i)   Heat cramps:
    - (a)   Pains develop in heavily exercising muscles in hot weather.
  - (ii)   Heat exhaustion:
    - (a)   Thirst, cramps, headache, vertigo, anorexia, nausea and vomiting occur;
    - (b)   The patient is flushed and sweating with rectal temperature 38°–39°C;
    - (c)   Tachycardia and orthostatic hypotension occur from dehydration.

(2) Severe heat illness with failure of thermoregulatory mechanisms:
  - (i)   Heat stroke:
    - (a)   Profuse sweating occurs in 50%, headache, vomiting and diarrhoea progressing to aggressive or bizarre behaviour, collapse, seizures and coma;
    - (b)   The rectal temperature is over 40°C.
    - (c)   The patient is flushed, tachypnoeic, tachycardic and hypotense. Muscle rigidity, transient hemiplegia, dilated pupils and disseminated intravascular coagulation all occur.

MANAGEMENT

(1) Heat cramps:
  - (i)   Rest in a cool environment and replace fluid orally with added salt or give 1 litre normal saline i.v.
  - (ii)   The patient is usually able to go home.
(2) Heat exhaustion:
  - (i)   Rest in a cool environment and give up to 3 litres cooled normal saline i.v.
  - (ii)   Cool the patient with tepid sponging and fanning.
  - (iii) Refer the patient to the medical team particularly when elderly or if orthostatic hypotension persists.

(3) Heat stroke:
    (i)   Give oxygen and attach an ECG monitor and pulse oximeter. Aim for an oxygen saturation above 94%.
    (ii)   Commence urgent cooling with tepid sponging, fans and cold packs to the groin and axillae until the temperature is less than 38.5°C.
    (iii) Gain intravenous access and send blood for FBC, coagulation profile, U&E, blood sugar, LFTs, creatine phosphokinase and check the blood gases.
    (iv) Give 1 litre cooled 4% dextrose 0.18% normal saline over 20 min then according to the blood pressure, U&E and urine output following bladder catheterisation.
    (v)   Give diazepam (Diazemuls) 5–10 mg i.v. for fits and chlorpromazine 25 mg i.v. to suppress shivering if the rate of cooling is inadequate. Endotracheal intubation is usually necessary.
    (vi) Refer the patient to the medical team for admission to ITU.

HYPOTHERMIA

This is present when the core temperature drops to less than 35°C (95°F). Mild hypothermia is classified as 32°–35°C, moderate 30°–32°C and severe hypothermia less than 30°C.

DIAGNOSIS

(1) Hypothermia is predisposed to in the following:
    (i)   elderly patients or babies;
    (ii)   unconscious patients or patients who have taken sedative drugs, especially alcohol;
    (iii) exposure to low air temperatures, particularly if there was associated wind and rain;
    (iv) exposure in cold water;
    (v)   endocrine disorders such as myxoedema or hypopituitary coma.

(2) Mild hypothermia causes lethargy, shivering and tachypnoea. Moderate hypothermia causes bradycardia, hypotension, bradypnoea, confusion and absent shivering.

(3) In severe hypothermia, the patient is comatose and may appear dead with an undetectable pulse, absent reflexes and fixed pupils.

(4) ECG changes include low voltage complexes, bradycardia, prolonged QT interval and a slurred notching of the terminal portion of the QRS complex — the J wave.

MANAGEMENT

(1) Record the core temperature rectally with a low-reading thermometer, or using a tympanic membrane device.

(2) Give high-dose oxygen which should be warmed and humidified if the core temperature is 32°C or less. Avoid endotracheal intubation if possible, as this may precipitate a cardiac arrhythmia.

(3) Cover the patient in warmed woollen blankets and layers of polythene. Warm the room air and minimise handling, aiming for a core temperature rise of 0.5°C per hour in the elderly, up to 1°C per hour in younger patients.

(4) Take blood for U&E, blood sugar and amylase as rarely pancreatitis may be associated.

(5) Check the blood gases to assess the degree of acidosis, but remember to inform the laboratory of the patient's temperature.

(6) Give intravenous fluids cautiously through a warming device. Pulmonary oedema may be precipitated by excessive fluid administration.

(7) Beware too rapid rewarming, as vasodilatation occurs causing hypotension, a further fall in temperature and ventricular fibrillation resistant to therapy.

(8) If a cardiac arrest occurs in a hypothermic patient:

    (i)   Commence cardiac massage and deliver three DC shocks, whilst a skilled doctor passes an endotracheal tube. Use warmed, humidified oxygen.

    (ii)   Bretylium may be more effective for VF than lignocaine.

   (iii) Continue resuscitation attempts until the core temperature rises to at least 32°C or until a senior doctor advises to the contrary.

      (a) This may involve a prolonged period of time when aggressive measures such as thoracotomy, mediastinal rewarming and internal defibrillation must be resorted to.

      (b) Other possible measures include peritoneal dialysis with warmed fluid or cardiopulmonary bypass, which is the method of choice when available.

      (c) Severe hyperkalaemia may be a useful prognostic indicator in hypothermic cardiac arrest to predict when aggressive resuscitation measures will not succeed.[5]

Note: with elderly, debilitated or deprived patients, remember to determine the predisposing factors to hypothermia before considering their discharge home, to prevent recurrence.

NEAR DROWNING

DIAGNOSIS

(1) The initial difference between sea water (hypertonic) and fresh water (hypotonic) near drowning is of little clinical significance, as only small amounts of fluid may have been aspirated.

(2) Consider other more relevant factors:

    (i)   Preceding injury, especially to the cervical spine in diving accidents.

    (ii) Sudden prior illness such as a myocardial infarction, cerebrovascular accident or epileptic fit that may have led to the drowning.

    (iii) Associated alcohol or drug use.

    (iv) Hypothermia.

(3) The presence of lung crackles indicates likely inhalation of water.

MANAGEMENT

(1) Commence cardiopulmonary resuscitation if the patient has no detectable cardiac output or is not breathing, taking due care for any possible neck injury. Prolonged resuscitation efforts may be successful, particularly if there was rapid associated hypothermia.

(2) Otherwise, give high-dose oxygen and measure the rectal temperature. Rewarm the patient if the core temperature is low (see page 81). Attach a cardiac monitor and pulse oximeter to the patient. Aim for an oxygen saturation above 94%.

(3) Check U&E, blood sugar, blood gases, CXR and ECG.

(4) Call the anaesthetist to intubate the patient if they are unconscious or develop respiratory failure with a PaO_2 less than 10 kPa on 50% oxygen, or a rising $PaCO_2$ above 7.5 kPa.

(5) Refer all patients to the medical team for admission. Delayed adult respiratory distress syndrome may develop from 6–48 h after submersion ('secondary drowning').

SPORTS (SCUBA) DIVING ACCIDENTS

The two main groups of accidents are decompression sickness and barotrauma.

DECOMPRESSION SICKNESS (CAISSON DISEASE)

This is due to inert nitrogen gas absorbed under pressure through the lungs becoming liberated throughout the body.

DIAGNOSIS

(1) Symptoms occur from several minutes up to 48 h after diving.

(2) Type 1 or mild:

(i)   Joint pain occurs, usually in a large joint such as the elbow or shoulder that may migrate and ranges from a dull ache to crippling — 'the bends'. Unusual fatigue and malaise are common;

(ii)   Skin itching, marbling or scarlatiniform rashes;

(iii) Painful lymphadenopathy and local oedema.

(3) Type 2 or serious:

(i)   Central nervous system involvement causes:

(a) Motor and sensory losses, personality disorder and seizures;

(b) Labyrinthine damage with deafness, tinnitus, nystagmus, vertigo and nausea — 'the staggers';

(c) Hemiplegia, paraplegia and urinary retention.

(ii)   Cardiopulmonary involvement causes retrosternal or pleuritic pain, dyspnoea, cough and haemoptysis — 'the chokes'. This can progress to respiratory failure and hypotension.

MANAGEMENT

(1) Give the patient 100% oxygen by tight-fitting face mask with reservoir bag.

(2) Gain intravenous access and commence normal saline rehydration.

(3) Give diazepam (Diazemuls) 5 mg i.v. for fits. This may also be used for severe labyrinthine disturbance after discussion with a diving medicine unit.

(4) Do not give strong analgesics, particularly opiates, as they mask symptoms.

(5) Refer every patient however strange their symptoms to a diving medicine unit:

(i)   Provide information about any dive in the preceding 48 h, the depth and duration and time of symptoms.

(ii)   Advice on diagnosis and arrangements for treatment are available from the following diving medicine units:

(a) Royal Navy, Portsmouth: Telephone 01705 818888.

(b) Aberdeen: Telephone 01224 681818.

(c) Co. Armagh: Telephone 01762 336711.

BAROTRAUMA

DIAGNOSIS

(1) Middle ear barotrauma:
   (i)   Local pain, sometimes with bleeding from the ear occurs associated with conductive deafness if the drum ruptures.
   (ii) The tympanic membrane appears reddened or may rupture.
(2) Inner ear barotrauma:
   (i)   Vertigo, tinnitus and sensorineural deafness occur due to a perilymph fistula, which mimick labyrinthine decompression sickness (see page 85).
(3) Sinus barotrauma:
   (i)   Local pain occurs over the maxillary and frontal sinus sometimes associated with bleeding.
(4) Dental barotrauma:
   (i)   Pain occurs in or around fillings or carious teeth.
(5) Pulmonary barotrauma:
   This is the most serious form of barotrauma causing:
   (i)   Surgical emphysema or pneumothorax associated with chest pain and dyspnoea;
   (ii) Arterial gas embolus affecting:
      (a) the coronary circulation with cardiac pain, arrhythmia and cardiac arrest;
      (b) the cerebral circulation with sudden onset of neurological symptoms just before or within 5 min of surfacing (without the delay seen in decompression sickness);
      (c) any neurological symptom or sign may occur from confusion to fits or coma and may fluctuate.

MANAGEMENT

(1) Middle ear barotrauma:
   (i)   Give an analgesic such as paracetamol 500 mg and codeine phosphate 8 mg (co-codamol) and an antibiotic such as amoxycillin 500 mg orally t.d.s. for 5 days.

    (ii)   Refer the patient to the next ENT clinic and ban further diving until the drum is fully healed.

(2) Inner ear barotrauma should be discussed immediately with a diving medicine unit as labyrinthine decompression sickness is a possible alternative diagnosis.

(3) Sinus and dental barotrauma require an analgesic such as paracetamol 500 mg and codeine phosphate 8 mg (co-codamol).

(4) Pulmonary barotrauma:

    (i)   Give oxygen and perform a CXR. Insert an intercostal drain if a significant pneumothorax is present (see page 24).

    (ii)   If arterial gas embolus is suspected:

        (a)   Keep the patient horizontal on their left side (not head down as this raises intracranial pressure),

        (b)   Give 100% oxygen by tight-fitting face mask with reservoir bag;

        (c)   Gain intravenous access and commence normal saline rehydration;

        (d)   Give diazepam (Diazemuls) 5 mg i.v. for fits;

        (e)   Refer the patient immediately to a diving medicine unit, even after apparent recovery as delayed deterioration can occur (see page 85 for telephone contact numbers).

VENOMOUS BITES AND STINGS

These are exceedingly rare in Britain, but may present following an altercation with an exotic pet or in zoo handlers and herpetologists. Specialist advice is available from the following centres:

National Poisons Information Service, London   0171 635 9191

Liverpool School of Tropical Medicine   0151 708 9393

as well as the other Poisons Information Centres (see page 67).

SNAKE BITES

DIAGNOSIS

(1) The adder is the only naturally occurring venomous snake in the UK.

(2) Immediate pain or swelling within hours indicate envenomation. However, under 50% of bites are associated with envenomation and occasionally systemic poisoning may occur with no local reaction.

(3) Systemic envenomation causes vomiting, abdominal pain and diarrhoea. Transient hypotension and coma may occur early, although the hypotension may persist in severe cases.

MANAGEMENT

(1) Reassure the patient, apply a firm bandage proximal to the bite, immobilise the dependent limb and transport all patients rapidly to hospital.

(2) Gain intravenous access and send blood for FBC, clotting screen, U&E and monitor the ECG. Give tetanus prophylaxis.

(3) Zagreb antivenom is available for adder envenomation.
  (i) This is indicated for:
    (a) hypotension;
    (b) bleeding;
    (c) ECG changes;
    (d) leucocytosis over $20\,000/mm^3$;
    (e) extending limb swelling, within 2 h of the bite.
  (ii) Two ampoules are added to normal saline 100 ml and infused at 1 ml/min initially.
  (iii) Adrenaline must be immediately available for hypersensitivity reactions.

(4) Refer all patients to the medical team for admission, even in the absence of any symptoms or signs.

MARINE ENVENOMATION

DIAGNOSIS

Several hazardous marine animals are found in UK coastal waters, including the following.
(1) Jellyfish:
    (i)   Sea nettle, compass, Portuguese man-of-war.
    (ii)   These cause burning local pain and oedema, with occasional systemic symptoms.
(2) Poisonous fish:
    (i)   Sting ray, lesser weever.
    (ii)   These cause extreme local pain and oedema, with various systemic effects including diarrhoea, respiratory depression and hypotension.
(3) Sea urchins:
    (i)   Injury is caused by the many tiny spines that may break off and enter joint cavities, or the deep palmar or plantar spaces.
    (ii)   There is excruciating local pain and oedema, with systemic effects including cardiorespiratory failure.

MANAGEMENT

(1) Use supportive measures including oxygen, analgesics and fluid replacement.
(2) Rinse jellyfish wounds with sea water, remove adherent tentacles and prevent further nematocyst discharge with acetic acid (vinegar).
(3) Poisonous fish and sea urchin wounds require:
    (i)   Pain relief by immersion in hot water or using a local anaesthetic block, followed by exploration, irrigation and debridement as necessary.
    (ii)   Tetanus prophylaxis and an antibiotic such as co-trimoxazole two tablets orally b.d. if there is extensive tissue damage.

BEE AND WASP STINGS

DIAGNOSIS

(1) There are more deaths in Britain and the USA from anaphylaxis following a bee or wasp sting than from all the other venomous bites and stings put together.

(2) Local pain predominates and may be followed by a severe anaphylactic reaction causing facial oedema, abdominal and back pain, difficulty in breathing, hypotension and collapse.

MANAGEMENT

(1) Remove bee stings by scraping out the sting with a knife without squeezing.

(2) Treat anaphylaxis with 0.3–0.5 ml of 1 in 1000 adrenaline i.m. or 1 in 10 000 adrenaline 0.75–1.5 µg/kg i.e. 50–100 µg or 0.5–1.0 ml for a 70-kg patient given slowly i.v. if circulatory collapse supervenes.

(3) Other measures include oxygen, airway management, hydrocortisone and chlorpheniramine (see page 107).

(4) Patients prone to anaphylaxis from bee or wasp stings should carry an adrenaline inhaler (Medihaler-epi) or a pre-filled adrenaline syringe at all times.

DISEASES IMPORTED FROM ABROAD

Patients who have been travelling outside the UK should be asked specifically about the time, place and type of travel. They should also be asked how much time they spent in each foreign country and how long they have been back in the UK.

Enquire about malaria prophylaxis and whether it was taken for 4 weeks after leaving the malarial zone, and about immunisations before going abroad.

Advice is always available in the UK from:

Hospital for Tropical Diseases, London	0171 387 4411
Liverpool School of Tropical Medicine	0151 708 9393
Communicable Diseases (Scotland) Unit	0141 946 7120
Recorded advice for travellers	01891 600350

Note: The DoH has issued a booklet 'Health Advice for Travellers' (code: T4), which is available by telephoning 0800 555 777. It contains country-by-country immunisation requirements, and details of health insurance and reciprocal agreements.

COMMON IMPORTED DISEASES OF TRAVELLERS

Many of these diseases are endemic in the UK but are more frequently contracted abroad. They are considered under the following headings:

(1) Human immunodeficiency virus (HIV) infection.
(2) Gastrointestinal tract infections:
    (i)   *Escherichia coli* gastroenteritis;
    (ii)   *Salmonella* and *Shigella gastroenteritis*;
    (iii) *Campylobacter* enteritis;
    (iv) giardiasis;
    (v)   amoebiasis.
(3) Helminth infections:
    (i)   schistosomiasis;
    (ii)   roundworm infection;
    (iii) tapeworm infection.
(4) Malaria.
(5) Typhoid.
(6) Viral hepatitis:
    (i)   hepatitis A;
    (ii)   hepatitis B;
    (iii) hepatitis C, D or E.

HUMAN IMMUNODEFICIENCY VIRUS (HIV) INFECTION

DIAGNOSIS

(1) Casual sexual intercourse, intravenous drug use and blood transfusion in countries with high carrier rates of HIV will expose the patient to infection.

(2) Assessment and diagnosis require a thorough clinical and laboratory appraisal. HIV testing in the A & E department is inappropriate as skilled counselling and follow-up are not available.

(3) Moreover, relying on a single serum test for HIV to exclude infection is unwise as:
   (i)   Occasional false positives occur;
   (ii) False negatives occur in those infected due to:
         (a) early infection;
         (b) lack of seroconversion in the first 4 months;
         (c) infection with HIV-2 when laboratory testing is for HIV-1 alone (most test for both).

MANAGEMENT

(1) All patients should be referred to the appropriate hospital outpatient clinic that provides a specialist screening service (see page 113 on acquired immune deficiency syndrome).

GASTROINTESTINAL TRACT INFECTION

DIAGNOSIS

(1) 'Traveller's diarrhoea' is most often due to enterotoxigenic *E. coli*, which is usually self-limiting over 2–5 days causing watery stools and occasionally vomiting. Fever is not a feature.

(2) *Salmonella* and *Shigella* infections tend to cause fever, diarrhoea (which may be bloodstained), vomiting and abdominal pain.

(3) *Campylobacter* infection presents with colicky abdominal pain that may precede the onset of diarrhoea, which is watery and offensive and sometimes blood-stained.

(4) Giardiasis causes acute watery diarrhoea which often persists beyond 10 days. Chronic infection may eventually cause malabsorption with steatorrhoea.

(5) Amoebiasis may also cause a chronic, recurrent diarrhoea, with stools containing blood and mucus.

(6) The most important feature in all cases is to assess the patient for dehydration. Dehydration causes thirst, lassitude, dry lax skin, tachycardia, postural hypotension leading to oliguria, confusion and coma.

MANAGEMENT

(1) In all dehydrated and febrile or toxic patients, send blood for FBC, U&E, blood culture and commence an intravenous infusion of normal saline.

(2) Refer the patient to the medical team.

(3) Other patients may be allowed home and encouraged to drink plenty of fluid. Alternatively, give the patient an oral glucose and electrolyte solution such as Dioralyte or Rehidrat, or simply advise him/her to add half a teaspoon of salt and 6 teaspoons of sugar to a litre of water.

(4) If symptoms persist, ask the patient to return within 24–48 h:

    (i)   Send stools for microscopy and culture then.

    (ii)   Give an antimotility agent such as loperamide 4 mg initially, followed by 2 mg after each loose stool to a maximum of 16 mg/day.

    (iii) Consider empirical treatment for moderate to severe diarrhoea with ciprofloxacin 500 mg orally b.d. for 3 days (not in children).

    (iv) If giardia is suspected, give tinidazole 2 g orally once.

    (v)   Arrange follow-up in medical outpatients or by the local general practitioner.

HELMINTH INFECTION

DIAGNOSIS

(1) Schistosomiasis rarely presents acutely, but should be suspected in cases from endemic areas presenting with fever and diarrhoea associated with eosinophilia, or in cases with painless terminal haematuria or obstructive uropathy.

(2) Roundworm infection is discovered when the adult worm is passed in the stool, although occasionally allergic pneumonitis, abdominal pain or urticaria occur.

(3) Tapeworm infection usually presents with lassitude, weight loss and anaemia.

MALARIA

DIAGNOSIS

(1) The patient usually presents within 4 weeks of returning from a malarious area with fever, rigors, nausea, vomiting, diarrhoea and headache. Hepatosplenomegaly is common.

(2) However, symptoms may occur months or even years later due to release of parasites from the exoerythrocytic phase in the liver (this does not occur in falciparum malaria).

(3) Falciparum malaria is the most dangerous form and may prove rapidly fatal. Most cases are imported from sub-Saharan Africa, South East Asia, the Amazon basin and Oceania.

    (i)   Large numbers of destroyed red cells affect the capillary circulation leading to damage to the brain, kidneys, liver, heart, gastrointestinal tract and lungs.

    (ii) Abrupt onset of encephalopathy with headache, confusion, fits and coma may occur known as cerebral malaria.

    (iii) Other presentations include an influenza-like illness, diarrhoea and vomiting, jaundice, acute

renal failure, acute respiratory distress, arthralgia, postural hypotension or shock, progressive anaemia and thrombocytopenia.
(iv)   The patient may not appear ill in the first few days, but nonimmune patients may then deteriorate rapidly over a few hours and die.

MANAGEMENT

(1) Send a thick and thin film for malarial parasites for every patient returning from abroad with fever and any of the above symptoms or signs. Also send a FBC, U&E and blood culture.
(2) Falciparum malaria is a medical emergency requiring prompt referral to the medical team for oral or intravenous quinine therapy, as most imported cases are chloroquine resistant.
(3) Other types of malaria should also be referred to the medical team, although some cases will be treated as outpatients.
(4) Ask patients with negative films, but a suggestive history to return for repeat blood films if symptoms persist. Inform the general practitioner of the possibility of malaria by telephone and a letter.
(i)   However, if falciparum malaria is likely, admit the patient immediately and begin treatment, if necessary before the blood results are available.

TYPHOID

DIAGNOSIS

(1) The incubation period is up to 3 weeks, with initial symptoms of malaise, headache, fever, dry cough and constipation in the first week.
(2) The illness may progress to abdominal distension and pain associated with diarrhoea, splenomegaly, bronchitis, confusion or coma and rarely a characteristic crop of fine rose-pink macules on the trunk.

(3) In the first week, blood cultures are positive in up to 90%, whereas in the second week stool culture becomes positive in 75% and urine culture in 25%.

MANAGEMENT

(1) Always send a blood culture in all suspected cases and a FBC that may show a leucopenia with a relative lympho-cytosis.
(2) Refer all cases to the medical team for ciprofloxacin orally or intravenously.
(3) Late cases should have stool and urine cultures sent as well.

VIRAL HEPATITIS

See page 188.

SICKLE CELL CRISES

DIAGNOSIS

(1) These occur in West Indians, Africans and rarely in Mediterraneans.
(2) The patient often knows his or her diagnosis and recognises an attack.
(3) Precipitating events include infection, dehydration, anaesthesia and cold.
(4) Two main types of crisis are seen:
    (i) *Vaso-occlusive crisis*. This provokes severe pain from local tissue infarction in the chest, abdomen, spine, large joint or bone.
    (ii) *Anaemic crisis*.
        (a) Sequestration: sudden painful enlargement of the liver and spleen presenting with cardio-vascular collapse.

(b) Haemolytic: massive haemolysis with a reticulocytosis, low haptoglobins and high indirect bilirubin.

(c) Hypoplastic: severe bone marrow depression usually in children.

(d) Megaloblastic: anaemia due to folate deficiency.

MANAGEMENT

(1) Check the haemoglobin. Most homozygous sicklers have haemoglobin levels of 7–10 g/dl, but the level will be much lower in an anaemic crisis.

(2) Confirm the sickle screen is positive, although this is not a quantitative test indicative of the severity of the crisis.

(3) Check U&E, blood sugar, LFTs, blood gases, MSU, CXR, ECG and blood cultures as indicated, and send a G&S.

(4) Give an analgesic such as morphine 5 mg i.v. and an antiemetic such as metoclopramide 10 mg i.v.

(5) Give intravenous fluids, but beware fluid overload causing pulmonary oedema.

(6) Give oxygen continuously, avoiding intermittent bursts, for hypoxaemia associated with pneumonia or vaso-occlusion.

(7) Refer all patients to the medical team.

Note: remember other problems that sicklers are prone to, include pulmonary infarct, cerebral infarct, osteomyelitis, aseptic necrosis of the head of the femur, dactylitis, cholecystitis, leg ulcers, vitreous haemorrhage and retinal detachment, and priapism.

ACUTE MONOARTHROPATHY

DIFFERENTIAL DIAGNOSIS

It is important to distinguish between:
(1) Trauma;
(2) Septic arthritis;

(3) Gout or pseudogout;
   and occasionally:
(4) Rheumatoid arthritis;
(5) Osteoarthritis.

TRAUMATIC ARTHRITIS

DIAGNOSIS

(1) Severe joint pain is usually associated with obvious trauma although occasionally the trauma is mild or even forgotten.
(2) X-rays are required but may not always demonstrate an obvious fracture (e.g. scaphoid or radial head) but may only show a joint effusion, or periosteal elevation as supporting evidence of fracture.
(3) If septic arthritis cannot be excluded, joint aspiration should be performed by the orthopaedic team which generally yields a haemorrhagic effusion, often with fat globules in cases of intra-articular fracture.

MANAGEMENT

Refer the patient to the orthopaedic team. Management varies according to the joint involved (see Section III, Orthopaedic Emergencies).

SEPTIC ARTHRITIS

DIAGNOSIS

(1) This occurs with penetrating trauma, which may be trivial e.g. a rose thorn or follows arthrocentesis. Most cases develop from haematogenous spread, predisposed to in patients with rheumatoid arthritis, sickle cell disease, intravenous drug abuse, debility, immunosuppression and disseminated meningococcal or gonococcal infection.
(2) There is localised pain, warmth and severely restricted movement with a less precipitate onset than with gout.

(3) X-rays will initially be normal, but subsequently show destruction of bone with loss of the joint space.

MANAGEMENT

(1) Check the temperature, pulse and BP; send blood for blood culture and FBC.
(2) Refer the patient immediately to the orthopaedic team for joint aspiration under sterile conditions, rest, intravenous antibiotics and repeated drainage.

GOUTY ARTHRITIS

DIAGNOSIS

(1) Gout is predisposed to by thiazide diuretic therapy, myeloproliferative disease (especially following treatment) and by dietary excess, alcohol and trauma.
(2) It is commonest in the metatarsophalangeal joint of the great toe or knee, sometimes with a precipitate onset waking the patient from sleep.
(3) Chronic cases may be associated with gouty tophi on the ear and around the joints, and recurrent acute attacks.
(4) The patient may be mildly pyrexial with a leucocytosis.
(5) The uric acid level is raised (over 0.4 mmol/l) but can be normal in an acute attack.
(6) Definitive diagnosis is by joint aspiration and polarising light microscopy showing strongly negative birefringent crystals.

MANAGEMENT

(1) In a known relapsing case, or if there is strong clinical suspicion of gout, give the patient diclofenac (Voltarol) 50 mg orally t.d.s. for 24 h, then 25 mg orally t.d.s. until the attack settles. Alternatively use naproxen (Naprosyn) 750 mg orally, followed by 250 mg orally t.d.s.
(2) Refer the patient back to the general practitioner or to medical outpatients.

(3) If septic arthritis cannot be excluded, refer the patient immediately to the orthopaedic team for joint aspiration.

PSEUDOGOUT

(1) This is much less common than gout, typically affecting the knee or wrist, and is associated with diabetes, osteoarthritis, hyperparathyroidism, haemochromatosis and many other rare conditions.
(2) X-ray may show chondrocalcinosis, and joint aspiration shows weakly positive birefringent crystals under polarising light microscopy.
(3) Treatment is as for acute gout, with referral back to the general practitioner or to medical outpatients for follow-up.

RHEUMATOID ARTHRITIS

DIAGNOSIS

(1) This occasionally presents as a monoarthritis, though generally it causes a symmetrical polyarthritis affecting the metacarpophalangeal and proximal interphalangeal joints in particular.
(2) Other joints affected include the knees, elbows and hips.
(3) X-rays initially show soft-tissue swelling only.
(4) Systemic involvement with malaise, weight loss, fever, pleurisy and pericarditis may occur.

MANAGEMENT

(1) If the patient is systemically unwell, refer to the medical team.
(2) If septic arthritis cannot be excluded, refer the patient to the orthopaedic team, remembering that rheumatoid arthritis actually predisposes to septic arthritis.
(3) Otherwise, check FBC, ESR, rheumatoid factor, ANF, and DNA antibodies and refer the patient to medical outpatients or the general practitioner.

(4) Commence a nonsteroidal anti-inflammatory agent such as diclofenac 50 mg orally t.d.s. or naproxen 500 mg orally b.d.

OSTEOARTHRITIS
DIAGNOSIS

(1) This usually presents as a polyarthritis of insidious onset typically affecting the distal interphalangeal joints.
(2) However, an acute monoarthritis with minimal systemic symptoms may be seen associated with marked joint crepitus.
(3) X-ray shows loss of joint space, osteophyte formation and bony cysts.

MANAGEMENT

(1) Refer the patient to the orthopaedic team if septic arthritis cannot be excluded.
(2) Otherwise, give the patient diclofenac 50 mg orally t.d.s. or naproxen 500 mg orally b.d. and refer back to the general practitioner.

ACUTE POLYARTHROPATHY

DIAGNOSIS

(1) There are many causes including:
    (i)   rheumatoid arthritis;
    (ii)   systemic lupus erythematosus;
    (iii)   osteoarthritis;
    (iv)   psoriatic arthritis;
    (v)   ankylosing spondylitis;
    (vi)   Reiter's syndrome;
    (vii)   viral illness e.g. hepatitis B or rubella;
    (viii) serum sickness;
    (ix)   ulcerative colitis, Crohn's disease, Behçet's disease etc.

MANAGEMENT

(1) Send blood for FBC, ESR, U&E, LFTs, uric acid, rheumatoid factor, ANF and DNA antibodies.
(2) If the patient is systemically unwell, refer to the medical team for bed rest, drug treatment and definitive diagnosis.
(3) Otherwise, commence a nonsteroidal anti-inflammatory agent such as diclofenac (Voltarol) 50 mg orally t.d.s. or naproxen 500 mg orally b.d. and refer the patient to medical or rheumatology outpatients.

NONARTICULAR RHEUMATISM

(1) Joint pain, swelling and tenderness mimicking arthritis can be due to inflammation of periarticular structures.
(2) Most patients may be treated with nonsteroidal anti-inflammatory analgesics such as diclofenac 50 mg orally t.d.s. or naproxen 500 mg orally b.d. and referred to outpatients or their general practitioner.
(3) Joint aspiration and steroid injection is best left to the experts, as complications such as septic arthritis and joint destruction could occur.
(4) Conditions in this category include:
   (i)   torticollis;
   (ii)   frozen shoulder;
   (iii)   supraspinatus tendinitis;
   (iv)   subacromial bursitis;
   (v)   tennis and golfer's elbow;
   (vi)   olecranon bursitis;
   (vii)   de Quervain's stenosing tenosynovitis;
   (viii) housemaid's knee.

TORTICOLLIS (WRY NECK)

DIAGNOSIS AND MANAGEMENT

(1) Ask the patient about recent trauma particularly in the elderly. Look specifically for local sepsis including tonsillitis, quinsy or a submandibular abscess.

(2) Exclude drug-induced dystonia due to metoclopramide, phenothiazines or haloperidol. Oculogyric crisis may also occur. Give benztropine (Cogentin) 1–2 mg i.v. followed by 2 mg orally once daily for 3 days if dystonia is likely.

(3) In the absence of the causes in (1) and (2) above use a counter-irritant spray such as PR Heat Spray locally, manipulate the neck into the neutral position and immobilise in a soft collar.

(4) Give an analgesic such as paracetamol 500 mg and codeine phosphate 8 mg (co-codamol) and return the patient to their general practitioner.

FROZEN SHOULDER

DIAGNOSIS AND MANAGEMENT

(1) This occurs spontaneously or following local trauma, or disuse of the arm after a fracture, CVA, myocardial infarction or even shingles. It is more common in the elderly.

(2) There is pain and loss of all movement.

(3) Encourage active shoulder movements following the above conditions, to prevent the condition occurring in the first place. Otherwise prescribe an anti-inflammatory analgesic and return the patient to their general practitioner.

(4) Physiotherapy may help but although the pain subsides, the loss of movement tends to persist for months or even years.

SUPRASPINATUS TENDINITIS

DIAGNOSIS AND MANAGEMENT

(1) This is one of the causes of the 'painful arc' between 60°–120° of shoulder abduction.

(2) X-ray may show calcification in the supraspinatus tendon.

(3) Give an anti-inflammatory analgesic, and consider referral to the orthopaedic clinic for aspiration and local steroid injection (or to the rheumatology clinic or general practitioner).

SUBACROMIAL BURSITIS

DIAGNOSIS AND MANAGEMENT

(1) This may be due to rupture of calcific material into the subacromial bursa again causing a 'painful arc', or constant severe pain.

(2) Treat as above.

TENNIS AND GOLFER'S ELBOW

DIAGNOSIS AND MANAGEMENT

(1) Tennis elbow causes pain over the lateral epicondyle of the humerus from a partial tear of the extensor origin of the forearm muscles used in repetitive movements (e.g. using a screwdriver or playing tennis).

(2) Advise the patient to avoid the activity causing the pain and to rest the arm; give an anti-inflammatory analgesic.

(3) If the pain is persistent, refer for local steroid injection.

(4) Golfer's elbow is a similar condition affecting the medial epicondyle and the flexor origin.

OLECRANON BURSITIS

DIAGNOSIS AND MANAGEMENT

(1) Painful swelling of this bursa is due to trauma, gout or sepsis.

(2) Aspiration should be performed under sterile conditions and fluid sent for culture and polarising light microscopy.

(3) The patient may require immediate referral for drainage of the bursa under anaesthesia if infection is suspected. Otherwise, refer the patient to orthopaedic outpatients for removal of the bursal sac.

DE QUERVAIN'S STENOSING TENOSYNOVITIS

DIAGNOSIS AND MANAGEMENT

(1) This causes tenderness over the radial styloid, a palpable nodule from thickening of the fibrous sheaths of the

abductor pollicis longus and extensor pollicis brevis tendons, and pain on moving the thumb.

(2) Treat by resting the thumb in a splint and by using an anti-inflammatory analgesic.

(3) This condition may require surgical release of the tendon sheaths if local injection of steroid fails.

HOUSEMAID'S KNEE

DIAGNOSIS AND MANAGEMENT

(1) This is a prepatellar bursitis due to friction, or occasionally infection.

(2) Treat by giving an anti-inflammatory analgesic, avoiding further trauma and, if necessary, by aspiration and steroid injection by the general practitioner or outpatient clinic (orthopaedic or rheumatology).

(3) If infection is suspected, refer the patient to the orthopaedic team.

ALLERGIC OR IMMUNOLOGICAL CONDITIONS

The following conditions may present ranging from socially inconvenient to imminently life threatening:

(1) urticaria;
(2) angioedema;
(3) anaphylaxis.

URTICARIA (HIVES)

DIAGNOSIS

(1) Itchy, oedematous, transient skin swellings are seen, which may occur in crops lasting several hours.

(2) Causes are many, including:
   (i)   Foods — shellfish, eggs, nuts, strawberries, chocolate.
   (ii) Drugs — penicillin, sulphonamide, aspirin, NSAID, codeine, morphine.

- (iii) Insect stings, animals, parasitic infections (children).
- (iv) Physical — cold, heat, sun, pressure, exercise.
- (v) Systemic illness — neoplasm, vasculitis, viral.
- (vi) Idiopathic (over 90% of chronic cases).

MANAGEMENT

- (1) Give the patient an H_1 antagonist such as terfenadine (Triludan) 60 mg orally b.d. This is not sedating, unlike chlorpheniramine (Piriton).
  - (i) Refractory cases may respond to the addition of an H_2 antagonist such as ranitidine 150 mg orally b.d.
- (2) Attempt to identify the likely cause from the recent history. Most reactions occur within minutes but may be delayed up to 24 h.

ANGIOEDEMA

DIAGNOSIS

- (1) An urticarial reaction involving the deep tissues of the face, eyelids, lips, tongue and occasionally the larynx often without pruritus.
- (2) The causes are as for urticaria, especially aspirin or a bee sting.
- (3) It may cause facial, lip and tongue swelling, progressing to laryngeal oedema with hoarseness, dysphagia and stridor.
- (4) A rare autosomal dominant hereditary form is due to C1 esterase inhibitor deficiency. A family history of attacks often following minor trauma and recurrent abdominal pain are suggestive.

MANAGEMENT

- (1) Commence high-dose oxygen and attach a cardiac monitor and pulse oximeter to the patient. Aim for an oxygen saturation above 94%.

(2) Give 1 in 1000 adrenaline 0.3–0.5 ml (0.3–0.5 mg) i.m. repeated as necessary.
(3) Give chlorpheniramine 10 mg i.v. but beware of sedation, hypotension and acute confusion.
(4) Refer the patient to the medical team for observation for at least 12 h, as relapse may occur.
(5) If airway obstruction persists, call the anaesthetist urgently and be prepared to intubate.
(6) Hereditary angioedema responds poorly to adrenaline and requires urgent fresh frozen plasma.

ANAPHYLAXIS

DIAGNOSIS

(1) An immunologically mediated systemic illness that may rapidly follow drug ingestion, particularly parenteral penicillin, a bee or wasp sting and food such as nuts and shellfish.
   (i)   An anaphylactoid reaction is a clinically identical syndrome most commonly following radio-contrast media or aspirin and other nonsteroidal anti-inflammatory drug exposure, which is not triggered by IgE antibody and therefore does not necessarily require previous exposure.[6]
(2) Respiratory manifestations:
   (i)   rhinitis;
   (ii)   laryngeal oedema and laryngeal obstruction;
   (iii) bronchospasm.
(3) Cardiovascular manifestations:
   (i)   tachycardia;
   (ii)   hypotension;
   (iii) circulatory collapse.
(4) Other manifestations:
   (i)   erythema;
   (ii)   local or widespread urticaria;
   (iii) angioedema;
   (iv)   headache;
   (v)   nausea, vomiting or diarrhoea;
   (vi)   joint pains and back pain.

MANAGEMENT

(1) Give high dose oxygen via a face mask, attach a cardiac monitor and pulse oximeter to the patient. Aim for an oxygen saturation above 94%.

(2) *Laryngeal oedema and wheeze*:

    (i) Give 0.3–0.5 ml of 1 in 1000 adrenaline i.m. immediately.

    (ii) Give hydrocortisone 200 mg i.v. and nebulised salbutamol 5 mg. Consider aminophylline 5 mg/kg i.v. over 20 min for persistent wheeze (providing the patient is not already taking oral theophylline).

(3) *Shock and circulatory collapse*:

    (i) Give 0.3–0.5 ml of 1 in 1000 adrenaline (0.3–0.5 mg) i.m. immediately, repeated every 5–10 min until improvement occurs.

    (ii) Give a bolus of polygeline (Haemaccel) 10–20 ml/kg i.v.

    (iii) Change to 1 in 10 000 adrenaline 0.75–1.5 µg/kg intravenously, i.e. 50–100 µg or 0.5–1.0 ml for a 70 kg patient if circulatory collapse persists.

(4) Additional second-line measures include:

    (i) Chlorpheniramine 10 mg i.v.;

    (ii) Hydrocortisone 200 mg i.v. (if not already given);

    (iii) Cimetidine 300 mg i.v. slowly for refractory hypotension;

    (iv) Glucagon 1 mg i.v. repeated as necessary, for patients on beta blockers resistant to the above treatment.

(5) Refer all patients to the medical team for admission. Up to 20% will relapse requiring further urgent treatment in the next 8–12 h.

SKIN DISORDERS

The vast majority of skin disorders are managed by general practitioners and the dermatology department, although some patients may present as emergencies with blistering or itching conditions. Malignant melanoma may also be seen.

BLISTERING CONDITIONS

DIAGNOSIS

(1) Common causes:
   (i)   Viral:
          (a) herpes zoster;
          (b) herpes simplex.
   (ii)   Impetigo;
   (iii) Scabies;
   (iv)   Insect bites and papular urticaria;
   (v)   Bullous eczema and pompholyx;
   (vi)   Drugs:
          (a) sulphonamides, penicillin, barbiturates.
(2) Less common causes:
   (i)   Erythema multiforme and Stevens–Johnson syndrome:
          (a) drug induced;
          (b) mycoplasma pneumonia;
          (c) herpes simplex.
   (ii)   Toxic epidermal necrolysis;
   (iii) Dermatitis herpetiformis;
   (iv)   Pemphigus and pemphigoid;
   (v)   Porphyria cutanea tarda.
(3) Rare causes:
   (i)   Congenital:
          (a) epidermolysis bullosa.

MANAGEMENT

(1) Refer patients with widespread or potentially life-threatening blistering immediately to the dermatology team or medical team.
   (i)   This should include patients with erythema multiforme, toxic epidermal necrolysis, pemphigus and pemphigoid.
(2) Otherwise give symptomatic treatment including:
   (i)   Antihistamine such as chlorpheniramine 4 mg orally q.d.s. if there is associated pruritus, with a warning about drowsiness.

(ii)   Antibiotics such as flucloxacillin 500 mg orally q.d.s. for secondary staphylococcal infection in herpes zoster, impetigo, insect bites and eczema or erythromycin 250 mg orally q.d.s. for patients allergic to penicillin.

(iii)   Parasiticidal preparation for scabies (see page 111).

(iv)   Antiviral agent such as acyclovir 200 mg orally five times a day for 5 days for severe herpes simplex or 800 mg orally five times a day for 7 days for severe herpes zoster.

(v)   Topical steroid antiseptic such as 0.1% betamethasone with 3% clioquinol (Betnovate C) cream three times daily for papular urticaria and bullous eczema.

(3) Return the patient to the care of their general practitioner.

PRURITUS (ITCHING CONDITIONS)

DIAGNOSIS

(1) Causes of pruritus with skin disease:
   (i)   Scabies, pediculosis, insect bites, parasites (roundworm);
   (ii)   Eczema;
   (iii)   Contact dermatitis;
   (iv)   Urticaria;
   (v)   Lichen planus;
   (vi)   Pityriasis rosea;
   (vii)   Dermatitis herpetiformis;
   (viii)   Drugs.

(2) Causes of pruritus without skin disease:
   (i)   Hepatic or biliary:
      (a) jaundice including primary biliary cirrhosis;
   (ii)   Chronic renal failure;
   (iii)   Haematological:
      (a) lymphoma;
      (b) polycythaemia rubra vera;

(iv) Endocrine:
    (a) myxoedema;
    (b) thyrotoxicosis;
(v) Carcinoma:
    (a) lung;
    (b) stomach;
(vi) Drugs.

MANAGEMENT

(1) Refer patients unable to sleep with intractable pruritus to the dermatology team or medical team.

(2) Otherwise give symptomatic treatment including:
  (i) Antipruritic drug:
    (a) chlorpheniramine 4 mg orally q.d.s. with a warning about drowsiness;
    (b) terfenadine, although non-sedating, does not cross the blood–brain barrier and is therefore ineffective for non-allergic pruritus.

  (ii) For scabies:
    (a) scabies is suggested by itch worse at night that does not involve the head, a close partner affected and finding burrows (often excoriated) in interdigital webs, around the genitalia or the nipples;
    (b) treat the patient and close contacts with 1% lindane or 0.5% malathion aqueous lotion over the whole body excluding the head, washed off after 24 h. All clothes are washed in addition;
    (c) warn the patient that although itching may persist it is no longer contagious;
    (d) advise the patient to attend a genitourinary medicine clinic to exclude an associated sexually transmitted disease.

  (iii) Cease any recent drug therapy considered causal including nonprescription.

  (iv) For urticaria — see page 105.

(3) Return the patient to the care of their general practitioner.

MALIGNANT MELANOMA

The incidence has doubled in many countries over the last decade.

DIAGNOSIS AND MANAGEMENT

(1) Revised checklist for suspected malignant melanoma:[7]
 (i)   Major signs:
  (a) change in size, e.g. an increase in size of a new or pre-existing cutaneous lesion;
  (b) change in shape, especially an irregular outline;
  (c) change in colour.
 (ii)   Minor signs:
  (a) inflammation;
  (b) crusting or bleeding;
  (c) sensory change including mild itch;
  (d) diameter 7 mm or more.
(2) Refer a patient with a pigmented lesion with any major sign urgently to the dermatology team.
(3) A patient with a pigmented lesion and a minor sign should also be referred although less than 50% will have a melanoma.
(4) Remember the commonest sites for a melanoma are on the back and on the legs.

SEXUALLY TRANSMITTED DISEASES

DIAGNOSIS

(1) Urethral discharge, dysuria, penile ulceration, warts and balanitis may present in males.
(2) Vaginal discharge, vaginal pruritus, ulceration, warts, menstrual irregularities and abdominal pain may present in females.

MANAGEMENT

(1) All sexually transmitted diseases require expert diagnosis, treatment, follow-up and partner contact tracing readily available in the Special Clinic (genitourinary medicine clinic).

(2) As many patients are reluctant to attend these clinics, explain carefully the local appointment system, what to expect and how to locate the clinic.
  (i) Advise males not to empty their bladder for at least 4 h prior to their attendance.

(3) Occasionally the patient will require hospital admission for the acute manifestations of AIDS, secondary syphilis, acute Reiter's syndrome, disseminated gonococcal infection, severe primary genital herpes or acute salpingitis
  (i) Genital herpes simplex infection:
    (a) treatment started early will reduce pain and shorten the acute attack;
    (b) give acyclovir 200 mg orally 5 times a day for five days;
    (c) this does not however influence the likelihood of later reactivation.

ACQUIRED IMMUNE DEFICIENCY SYNDROME (AIDS)

DIAGNOSIS

(1) This is caused by a lymphotropic retrovirus called human immunodeficiency virus (HIV). It is transmitted by sexual contact, syringe sharing in intravenous drug abusers, by blood transfusion and transplacentally.

(2) AIDS risk groups include:
  (i) Homosexual and bisexual males;
  (ii) Intravenous drug abusers;
  (iii) Haemophiliacs and transfusion recipients;

    (iv)   Heterosexual partners of HIV patients;

    (v)   Children of affected mothers.

(3) CDC classification of HIV infection (Centers for Disease Control and Prevention, Atlanta, Georgia USA) 1986:[8]

    (i)   Group 1: Acute infection.

    (ii)   Group 2: Asymptomatic infection.

    (iii)   Group 3: Persistent generalised lymphadenopathy (PGL).

    (iv)   Group 4: Symptomatic infection:

        (a)   subgroup A: nonspecific constitutional disease.

        (b)   subgroup B: neurological disease.

        (c)   subgroup C: secondary infectious diseases categories C1 and C2.

        (d)   subgroup D: secondary cancers.

        (e)   subgroup E: other conditions.

(4) A revised classification system for HIV infection and an expanded surveillance case definition for AIDS among adolescents and adults were published by the CDC in 1992:[9]

    (i)   These emphasise the clinical importance of the absolute CD4+ T-lymphocycte count or its percentage of the total lymphocyte count;

    (ii)   They are primarily intended for use in public health practice and have been utilised in the USA since 1993 for case reporting;

    (iii)   The original CDC 1986 system is still in common use and is discussed below, with the 1992 additions included.

(5) Presentation varies according to the disease group:

    (i)   Group 1: Acute infection.

        (a)   50%–70% of patients infected with HIV develop an acute illness with lethargy, fever, pharyngitis, myalgia, rash and lymphadenopathy about 2 weeks after exposure. Acute meningitis or encephalitis is occasionally seen.

        (b)   Although the patient is infectious, serology for HIV antibodies at this early stage will be negative.

   (ii)   Group 2: Asymptomatic infection.
- (a) Acute infection symptoms usually resolve by 3 weeks.
- (b) Infected patients seroconvert to HIV positive over the next 4 months, most within 2–12 weeks of exposure.
- (c) 50% of these patients will have fully developed AIDS by 10 years, with a near 100% mortality within 3 years of its development.

   (iii)   Group 3: Persistent generalised lymphadenopathy.
- (a) Enlarged nodes in two or more noncontiguous extra-inguinal sites for at least 3 months and not due to a disease other than HIV.
- (b) The patient is otherwise relatively well.

   (iv)   Group 4. Symptomatic infection.
- (a) Subgroup A: constitutional disease with persistent fever, unexplained weight loss of 10% body mass or diarrhoea for over 1 month.
- (b) Subgroup B: neurological disease including encephalopathy, myelopathy and peripheral neuropathy.
- (c) Subgroup C: secondary infectious diseases due to opportunistic infections including *Pneumocystis carinii* pneumonia, recurrent pneumonia, *Mycobacterium tuberculosis*, atypical mycobacteria, toxoplasmosis, cryptosporidiosis, strongyloidosis, cytomegalovirus, systemic candidiasis, cryptococcosis and many others.
- (d) Subgroup D: secondary cancers including Kaposi's sarcoma, high-grade nonHodgkin's lymphoma, primary lymphoma of the brain and invasive cervical cancer.
- (e) Subgroup E: other conditions such as the HIV wasting syndrome and chronic lymphoid interstitial pneumonitis.

(6) Thus, patients encountered in the A & E department with HIV will range from the asymptomatic carrier state

in the majority to nonspecific illness or acute problems as varied as collapse, respiratory failure, gastrointestinal bleeding, skin disorders, depression, dementia, stroke and coma.

MANAGEMENT

(1) Always maintain a high index of suspicion to identify the AIDS-risk patient, if necessary by direct questioning.

(2) However, consider all patients to be potentially infected and adopt Universal Precautions with every patient to prevent any disease transmission:

    (i)   Hands should always be washed before and after contact with patients.

    (ii)   Gloves should always be worn when handling blood specimens and body fluids.

    (iii) Disposable aprons should be worn if there is likely to be contamination of clothing (e.g. from bleeding), and face masks and goggles used if splashing is a possibility.

    (iv) Great care should be taken in handling needles or scalpel blades, particularly on disposal.

    (v)   Blood spills must be cleaned immediately with a suitable chlorine-based disinfectant.

(3) If the patient is acutely ill, refer him or her to the medical team in the usual way. Otherwise refer the patient to the genitourinary medicine Special Clinic or to the appropriate medical outpatient clinic.

Note: HIV antibody testing should not be offered on demand unless the patient has been fully counselled on the use and implications of a positive or negative test.

INOCULATION ACCIDENTS

INOCULATION ACCIDENTS WITH HIV RISK

If accidental inoculation of blood or infectious material from a suspected HIV antibody-positive patient occurs:

(1) Use a skin antiseptic such as 0.5% chlorhexidine in 70% alcohol and encourage bleeding by local venous occlusion.

(2) Take 10 ml clotted blood with consent from the injured person, and if possible 10 ml with consent from the source. Send for HIV testing.

(3) If the source is known to be HIV positive and massive exposure has occurred e.g. deep needlestick or laceration with blood inoculated, consider immediate zidovudine prophylaxis:

    (i)   Give zidovudine 200 mg orally 4-hourly;

    (ii)   Side effects include fever, headache, insomnia, anorexia, nausea and blood dyscrasias;

    (iii) Its use is controversial, and must be guided by hospital policy.

(4) Refer the injured person to Occupational Health for follow-up, advice and counselling. Report the incident to the senior member of the A & E staff and infection control officer.

(5) The risk of seroconversion following a needlestick injury with HIV-positive blood is less than 1 in 300.

(6) Consider the additional possibility of transmission of hepatitis B (see below) and the need for tetanus prophylaxis.

INOCULATION ACCIDENTS WITH HEPATITIS B RISK

(1) Wash the area with soap and water, dress the wound and give tetanus prophylaxis.

(2) Use Table 5 for recommendations for hepatitis B prophylaxis following percutaneous exposure.

(3) Refer the patient to Occupational Health for follow-up. Inform the senior A & E doctor and infection control officer.

(4) The risk of seroconversion in a nonimmunised person following a needlestick injury with HBV-positive blood is 1 in 5.

Table 5. Hepatitis B prophylaxis following percutaneous exposure

| Source | Exposed person | |
	Unvaccinated	Previously vaccinated with HB vaccine
HBsAg positive	(1) HBIG immediately (2) Initiate HB vaccine series	(1) Test exposed person for anti-HBs (2) If anti-HBs level inadequate, give HBIG immediately and booster HB vaccine
Known source: High risk of being HBsAg positive	(1) Initiate HB vaccine series (2) Test source for HBsAg and if positive, give exposed person HBIG in addition	(1) Test exposed person for anti-HBs and if level inadequate, test source for HBsAg (2) If source positive, treat as (2) above
Known source: Low risk of being HBsAg positive	Initiate HB vaccine series	Nothing required
Source unknown or untraceable	Initiate HB vaccine series	Nothing required

Key: HBsAg = Hepatitis B surface antigen
      Anti-HBs = Antibody to HBsAg
      HBIG = Hepatitis B immune globulin
      HB vaccine = Hepatitis B vaccine
From *MMWR;* (1985) **34**:331

THE ELDERLY PATIENT

(1) An increasing number of patients over the age of 65 attend A & E departments and pose unique problems of their own.

(2) These problems begin in the waiting area, where old people may become frightened or confused due to their inability to see, hear or move easily and understand instructions.

(3) Particular factors must always be considered before discharging an elderly patient. Ask yourself the following questions:

  (i) Can the patient walk safely with or without a stick?

  (ii) Can the patient get home safely and easily?

  (iii) Once home, can the patient cope with dressing, washing, using the toilet, shopping, cooking, cleaning or relaxing?

  (iv) Can the patient understand new or existing medication?

  (v) Can relatives or friends cope any more?

(4) If any answers to the above are 'no', do not discharge the patient until help has been sought from the following people. If necessary, keep the patient overnight to facilitate arrangements:

  (i) General practitioner:
    (a) the key person to coordinate the care of the patient at home;
    (b) always contact by telephone, as well as by letter.

  (ii) Social worker (hospital or community-based), who can offer:
    (a) home help;
    (b) 'meals on wheels';
    (c) lunch and recreational clubs;
    (d) voluntary visiting services;
    (e) laundry service;
    (f) chiropody service;
    (g) home adaptation service;

(h)   sheltered accommodation;

(i)   part III accommodation: to be eligible for part III accommodation, the patient must be ambulant (using a stick or frame if necessary), able to dress, wash and feed himself or herself, able to use a toilet, and should not be so confused as to require constant attention.

(iii)   District nursing service: this includes an evening and night nursing service.

(iv)   Health visitor.

(v)   Domiciliary physiotherapist or occupational therapist.

DISORDERED BEHAVIOUR IN THE ELDERLY

A breakdown in a patient's normal, socially acceptable behaviour can be classified into three broad categories:
 (1) Delirium (toxic confusional state);
 (2) Dementia (organic confusional state);
 (3) Depression (psychiatric confusional state).

DIAGNOSIS

(1) Delirium or toxic confusional state.

(i)   This includes clouding of consciousness and failure of recent memory and attention.

(ii)   It results in an acute confusional state with recent memory loss, associated with aggressive, restless behaviour and hallucinations, often worse at night.

(iii)   Causes are many, including:

(a)   Infection — pneumonia, UTI, cholecystitis, septicaemia.

(b)   Hypoxia — respiratory disease, heart failure, anaemia.

(c)   Cerebral ischaemia — TIA, stroke.

(d)   Cerebral lesion — haematoma, tumour, infection.

(e)   Iatrogenic — many drugs (remember poisoning, both accidental and deliberate), alcohol.

(f)   Vitamin deficiency — poor diet.

(g) Metabolic – including dehydration and electrolyte imbalance.

(h) Pain, cold, urinary retention, faecal impaction.

(2) Dementia or organic confusional state.

(i) This includes disorientation in place, time and person, abnormal or antisocial behaviour, short-term memory loss, loss of intellect and loss of insight.

(ii) The causes are many, although a definitive new diagnosis is seldom made in the A&E department.

(iii) However, if a known demented patient is brought into the A&E department with recent deterioration, the causes in 1 (iii) above should be sought.

(3) Depression or psychiatric confusional state.

(i) This includes difficulty in sleeping, demanding or withdrawn behaviour, hypochondriasis, a loss of self-interest and a sense of futility.

(ii) Suicide is a risk, particularly if the patient lives alone and is physically incapacitated or has made previous attempts at suicide.

MANAGEMENT

(1) A toxic confusional state and decompensated dementia require hospital admission (do not simply sedate).

(2) Depression and a high suicide risk require urgent referral to a psychiatrist and possible hospital admission.

FALLS IN THE ELDERLY

DIAGNOSIS

Two aspects must always be considered following a fall in the elderly:

(1) *The cause of the fall.*

(i) Accidental:

(a) obstacles in the home such as a trailing flex, the edge of a carpet, poor lighting and no hand rails.

    (ii)   Musculoskeletal:
- (a) arthritis;
- (b) obesity;
- (c) physical inactivity.

    (iii)   Visual failure:
- (a) cataracts;
- (b) senile macular degeneration;
- (c) glaucoma.

    (iv)   Sedating drugs:
- (a) benzodiazepines;
- (b) antihistamines;
- (c) psychotropics.

    (v)   Postural hypotension:
- (a) autonomic failure;
- (b) drug induced;
- (c) hyponatraemia.

    (vi)   Syncopal episode:
- (a) vertebrobasilar insufficiency;
- (b) cardiac arrhythmia, infarction, heart block.

    (vii) Cerebral disorder:
- (a) Parkinson's disease;
- (b) seizure;
- (c) stroke.

    (viii) Balance disorder: inner ear disease.

(2) *The result of the fall.*

    (i)   Fracture:
- (a) Colles';
- (b) neck of femur or pelvis;
- (c) skull;
- (d) ribs.

    (ii)   Hypothermia.

    (iii) Pressure sores, rhabdomyolysis.

    (iv) Hypostatic pneumonia.

    (v)   Loss of confidence and independence.

MANAGEMENT

(1) All falls in the elderly, particularly if recurrent, must be diagnosed and managed correctly, otherwise a fatal injury will eventually occur.

(2) Refer the patient to the medical or geriatric team for admission if acute care is needed or if there is any doubt about their ability to cope at home.

(3) Otherwise, refer to outpatients, physiotherapy, occupational therapy or social services and liaise closely with the general practitioner.

REFERENCES

1 European Resuscitation Council Basic Life Support Working Group (1993). Guidelines for basic life support. *British Medical Journal*; **306**:1587–1589.

2 European Resuscitation Council (1993). Adult advanced cardiac life support: the European Resuscitation Council guidelines 1992 (abridged). *British Medical Journal*; **306**:1589–1593.

3 Miller A.C., Harvey J.E. (1993). Guidelines for the management of spontaneous pneumothorax. *British Medical Journal*; **307**:114–116.

4 British Thoracic Society (1993). Guidelines for the management of asthma: a summary. *British Medical Journal*; **306**:776–782.

5 Keatinge W. R. (1991). Hypothermia: dead or alive? *British Medical Journal*; **302**:3–4.

6 Brown A.F.T. (1995). Anaphylactic shock: mechanisms and treatment. *Journal of Accident and Emergency Medicine*; **12**:89–100.

7 Mackie R.M. (1990). Clinical recognition of early invasive malignant melanoma. *British Medical Journal*; **301**:1005–1006.

8 CDC (1986). Classification system for human T-lymphotropic virus type III/lymphadenopathy-associated virus infections. *Morbidity and Mortality Weekly Report*; **35**:334–339.

9 CDC (1992). 1993 revised classification system for HIV infection and expanded surveillance case definition for AIDS among adolescents and adults. *Morbidity and Mortality Weekly Report*; **41** (RR-17):1–19.

SURGICAL EMERGENCIES

HEAD INJURY

The diagnosis and management of head injuries will be considered in two groups:
  (1) The seriously injured or unconscious head injury.
  (2) The conscious head injury.

THE SERIOUSLY INJURED OR UNCONSCIOUS HEAD INJURY

DIAGNOSIS

  (1) The head injury may be obvious from the history or on immediate examination.
  (2) The possibility of a head injury must be considered in every instance of coma or abnormal behaviour, in at-risk groups such as drunks and epileptics, nonaccidental injury in children, and in falls in the elderly.

MANAGEMENT

  (1) Clear the airway by sucking out any secretions, remove loose or broken dentures and insert an oropharyngeal airway. Give 100% oxygen by tight-fitting mask with reservoir bag.
  (2) Immobilise the cervical spine by applying a semi-rigid collar as up to 10% of patients with blunt head trauma have a concomitant neck injury.
    (i)   In addition, use sandbags on either side of the head taped to the forehead, unless the patient is excessively restless.
  (3) If the gag reflex is reduced or absent the patient requires intubating:
    (i)   Call the anaesthetist immediately to pass a cuffed endotracheal tube;
    (ii) Take great care to minimise neck movements by an assistant providing in-line manual immobilisation of the neck throughout.

(4) If the respirations are rapid or ineffectual, consider whether a tension pneumothorax (see page 137), open pneumothorax (see page 136), massive haemothorax (see page 150) or flail chest (see page 151) is responsible.

(5) Record the temperature, pulse, blood pressure and respirations, and attach an ECG monitor and pulse oximeter to the patient. Aim for an oxygen saturation above 94%.

(6) (i) Gain intravenous access and send blood for FBC, cross-match, glucose, U&E and save serum for a drug screen, in case alcohol or drug intoxication is subsequently suspected.

   (ii) Send arterial blood gases, recording the percentage of inspired oxygen being given at the time.

   (iii) Avoid excessive fluid administration if the patient is normotensive, as this may contribute to cerebral oedema.

(7) If the patient is hypotensive:

   (i) Search for associated injuries including chest, abdominal or pelvic bleeding, long-bone fracture and cardiac tamponade.

   (ii) Occasionally brisk scalp bleeding alone is found to be responsible, usually in children. Alternatively, cervical or high thoracic spinal cord injury with loss of sympathetic vascular tone may be the cause.

   (iii) Commence intravenous fluid administration to restore normotension using a plasma expander such as polygeline (Haemaccel).

(8) Record the level of consciousness using the Glasgow Coma Scale (GCS) score (Table 6):

   (i) A patient in coma has a score of 8 or less.

   (ii) A decrease in score of 2 or more points indicates significant deterioration.

   (iii) Repeated neurological examination including the Glasgow Coma Scale is essential for detecting and managing secondary brain damage.

(9) Treat the following complications immediately as they worsen existing cerebral damage:

Table 6. The Glasgow Coma Scale

		Score
Eye opening:	spontaneously	4
	to speech	3
	to pain	2
	none	1
Verbal response:	orientated	5
	confused	4
	inappropriate	3
	incomprehensible	2
	none	1
Motor response:	obeys commands	6
	localises pain	5
	withdraws (pain)	4
	flexion (pain)	3
	extension (pain)	2
	none	1

The maximum score is 15. Any reduction in the score indicates a deterioration in the level of consciousness.

(i)   Hypoxia: PaO_2 less than 9 kPa breathing air or 13 kPa on supplemental oxygen and hypercarbia with $PaCO_2$ over 6 kPa in the spontaneously breathing patient necessitate endotracheal intubation by the anaesthetist.

(ii) Seizures: give intravenous diazepam (Diazemuls) 5–10 mg in the adult, followed by phenytoin 15 mg/kg i.v. (see page 51).

(iii) Hypoglycaemia:
      (a) Check a Glucostix and if it is low, send a blood glucose to the laboratory and give 50 ml of 50% dextrose intravenously.
      (b) Remember this particularly if the patient has been drinking.

(iv) Pinpoint pupils:
      (a) Give naloxone 0.8–2 mg i.v.
      (b) If there is no response, this may indicate pontine or cerebellar damage.

(v)   Restless or aggressive behaviour:

     (a) Check the airway is still patent and high-dose oxygen is being delivered;

     (b) Repeat the BP, to look for hypotension;

     (c) Catheterise the bladder, and exclude a constricting bandage or tight cast.

  (vi) Gastric distension: pass a large-bore nasogastric tube, or orogastric tube if a basal skull or midface fracture is present.

(10) Perform a neurological examination including:

  (i) Conscious level: repeat the GCS record and look for any deterioration (decrease in score).

  (ii) Pupil size and reactions: look in particular for an unequal or dilating pupil indicating rising intracranial pressure.

  (iii) Eye movements and fundoscopy:

     (a) Intact eye movements are one indicator of brainstem function.

     (b) Fundoscopy may reveal papilloedema, subhyaloid haemorrhage or retinal detachment.

  (iv) The other cranial nerves: include examination of the corneal reflex, facial movements and the cough and gag reflexes.

  (v) Limb movements:

     (a) Assess for abnormal tone, weakness or loss of movement, or an asymmetric response to pain if the patient is unconscious.

     (b) Check the limb reflexes including the plantar responses.

(11) In the patient with a deteriorating level of consciousness or focal neurological signs, particularly a dilating pupil associated with bradycardia and hypertension:

  (i) Call the anaesthetist urgently to pass an endotracheal tube if not already positioned;

  (ii) Hyperventilate the patient to a $PaCO_2$ of 3.5–4.0 kPa in consultation with the neurosurgical team, who will also advise on the use of intravenous 20% mannitol 0.5–1 g/kg (2.5–5 ml/kg).

(12) Examine the scalp for bruising, lacerations and haematomas, and palpate for a deformity indicating a depressed fracture.

(13) Examine the face and mouth for signs of facial fracture or basal skull fracture:
  (i)   Basal skull fracture is indicated by:
    (a) Periorbital and subconjunctival haemorrhage.
    (b) Haemotympanum, external bleeding or CSF leak from the ear.
    (c) Mastoid bruising (Battle's sign) which may not appear for many hours.
    (d) Haemorrhage or CSF leakage from the nose.
    (e) Nasopharyngeal haemorrhage that may be profuse.
(14) Perform a head-to-toe assessment for other injuries of the neck, chest, back, limbs, abdomen and perineum including a rectal examination (loss of anal tone may indicate spinal cord damage).
(15) Request radiological examinations as follows:
  (i)   Lateral cervical spine:
    (a) This should *always* be performed in any unconscious head injury or in a suspected neck injury, combined with an anteroposterior and open-mouth view (for odontoid peg fracture) as well.
    (b) Make sure C1–C7/T1 are visualised, if necessary by traction on the shoulders.
  (ii)   Chest x-ray and pelvic x-ray in all multiply injured patients.
  (iii) Skull x-rays:
    (a) These are of minimal value in the early management of a major head injury if there is easy access to CT scanning and are never a substitute for carefully repeated neurological examination.
    (b) Look for a linear fracture, the double shadow of a depressed fracture, suture diastasis, an air–fluid level in a sinus, a traumatic aerocoele or shift of the pineal.
  (iv)   Do not request facial views or base-of-skull views at this stage.
(16) Obtain the history from the ambulance crew, police or

any witnesses of the circumstances and nature of the injury, observed loss of consciousness or subsequent epileptic fits.

(17) Obtain any other medical details if a relative or friend is available, of current medical or surgical conditions, drug therapy, allergies and previous head injury or epilepsy.

(18) If a compound or depressed skull fracture is found or intracranial air, give either ampicillin 1 g i.v. with sulphadiazine 1 g i.v. or ceftriaxone 1 g i.v. and tetanus prophylaxis.

(19) Refer all patients to the care of the surgical team. Obtain early neurosurgical advice and arrange a CT scan.

(20) Indications for CT head scan in general hospitals:[1]
    (i)   Confusion persisting after initial assessment and resuscitation;
    (ii) Unstable systemic state precluding transfer to neurosurgery;
    (iii) Full consciousness but with a skull fracture;
    (iv) Diagnosis uncertain.

(21) Indications for referral to a neurosurgical unit:[1]
    (i)   Without preliminary CT head scan:
        (a) Coma persisting after resuscitation;
        (b) Deteriorating consciousness or progressive focal neurological deficits;
        (c) Open injury: depressed fracture of vault or basal skull fracture;
        (d) Patient fulfils criteria for a CT scan in a general hospital when this cannot be performed within a reasonable time e.g. 3–4 h.
    (ii) After CT head scan in general hospitals:
        (a) Abnormal scan (ideally after neurosurgical opinion on images transferred electronically);
        (b) Scan considered normal but patient's progress unsatisfactory.

(22) It is essential that the patient's condition is stable and any associated injuries have been dealt with before transferring the patient.[2]
    (i)   The transport team should be suitably experienced and carry appropriate monitoring equipment.

THE CONSCIOUS HEAD INJURY

The aim is to differentiate patients requiring admission from those who could be allowed home.

DIAGNOSIS

(1) *History*. Enquire about:
   (i)   The nature and speed of impact.
   (ii) Subsequent loss of consciousness, drowsiness, vomiting or fits.
   (iii) The length of post-traumatic amnesia (PTA) from the time of injury to the time of the return of memory for consecutive events. It is often under-estimated.
        (a) Over 10 minutes PTA is significant.
   (iv) Associated alcohol or drug intoxication.
   (v)   Relevant medical conditions and drug therapy, including warfarin.

(2) *Examination*.
   (i)   Examine the scalp for bruising, lacerations or palpable fractures and haematomas.
   (ii) Assess the higher mental functions, including the level of consciousness using the GCS (see page 128).
   (iii) Check the pupil size and reactions, eye movements, cranial nerves and the limbs for later-alising neurological signs.
   (iv) Record the temperature, pulse, blood pressure and respirations.
   (v)   Exclude associated neck or other injuries.

(3) *X-ray*. Patients with the following conditions should have a skull x-ray, including an anteroposterior, lateral and a Towne's view (which visualises the occiput):
   (i)   Any loss of consciousness or significant PTA; history unknown or unreliable (e.g. under the influence of alcohol or drugs).
   (ii) High-speed injury, injury from a sharp or heavy object or a suspected penetrating injury.
   (iii) Deep scalp laceration, large haematoma or fracture suspected on palpation.

(iv) Focal neurological signs or impaired consciousness.
(v) Repeated vomiting or headache.
(vi) Cerebrospinal fluid or blood loss from the nose or ear.
(vii) Difficulty assessing the patient, e.g. children, the elderly or epileptic.

Note: with the increasing availability of CT scanning, most of the above patients should now proceed directly to a CT head scan.

MANAGEMENT

(1) Scalp lacerations should be thoroughly cleaned, the edges trimmed and any foreign bodies removed. They are then sutured in one layer using a monofilament synthetic material such as polyamide (Ethilon).
(2) Give tetanus prophylaxis according to the patient's immune status.
(3) *Admission.*
   (i) An adult patient who has a skull fracture but no impairment of consciousness has a 1 in 45 risk of developing a significant intracranial haematoma.[1]
   (ii) An adult patient in coma (GCS 8 or less) but with no skull fracture has a 1 in 27 risk of developing a significant intracranial haematoma, and with impaired consciousness but no skull fracture a 1 in 180 risk.[1]
   (iii) Therefore, refer any of the following to the surgical team for admission. Many patients will require a CT head scan and some even referral to a neurosurgical unit (see criteria on page 131).
      (a) skull fracture on x-ray;
      (b) impaired consciousness irrespective of the use of alcohol, or a history of unconsciousness of over 5 min;
      (c) repeated vomiting or persistent headache;
      (d) fits or focal CNS signs;
      (e) patient aged under 5 or over 50 years;

(f)   patient haemophiliac or on anticoagulants;

(g)   significant associated injuries.

(4) *Discharge.*

(i)   An adult who has no skull fracture and no impairment of consciousness has only a 1 in 7866 chance of developing a significant intracranial haematoma.[1]

(ii) The following patients may therefore be sent home, providing there is someone with them and home circumstances are suitable:

(a)   fully conscious and orientated;

(b)   no skull fracture;

(c)   no other significant injuries;

(d)   no fits nor focal neurological signs;

(e)   no persistent headache nor vomiting.

(iii) Each patient must be given a standard head injury warning card advising him or her to return if any complications develop within the next 24 h, such as confusion, drowsiness, seizure, visual disturbance, vomiting or persistent headache.

(5) *The remainder.* This leaves patients who have:

(i)   no one to accompany them;

(ii) poor home circumstances;

(iii) other significant injuries to the face or nose, etc.;

(iv) an unreliable history, particularly if under the influence of alcohol.

They should all be admitted to the short-stay ward for regular neurological observations.

(6) *Always remember*:

(i)   In the elderly, the cause of the original fall may have been a TIA, Stokes–Adams attack or other syncopal episode which requires diagnosis and management in its own right, in addition to the resultant head injury.

(ii) In children, a head injury may be due to nonaccidental injury (see page 274).

(iii) A skull fracture can occur without loss of consciousness, and conversely significant intracranial injury can be sustained without fracturing the skull, particularly in children.

MULTIPLE INJURIES

The management of the severely injured patient is best coordinated by adopting a standard routine for assessment as taught, for example, in advanced trauma life-support (ATLS) courses. This involves a rapid primary survey, resuscitation of vital functions, a detailed secondary survey and the initiation of definitive care.

(1) The primary survey identifies life-threatening conditions which are corrected immediately, as the respiratory and circulatory status are optimised in the resuscitation phase.

(2) The secondary survey commences after the primary survey is complete and the resuscitation phase underway:
  (i) A detailed head-to-toe examination is made;
  (ii) Initial x-rays are taken, bloods sent and procedures such as peritoneal lavage performed.

(3) Definitive care is the management of all the injuries identified including surgery, fracture stabilisation, hospital admission or the preparation for patient transfer, should this be necessary.

(4) Always call senior A & E staff for any multiple injury patient, so that they may organise an integrated team response incorporating anaesthetic, surgical and orthopaedic colleagues.

(5) Expect serious injuries in the following high-risk patients:
  (i) High speed impact, ejection or death of another vehicle occupant;
  (ii) Entrapment;
  (iii) Fall greater than 15 feet (5 metres);
  (iv) Motorcyclist or pedestrian struck;
  (v) Abnormal vital signs (systolic BP under 90 mmHg, GCS 12 or less, respiratory rate under 10 or over 29 per minute).

(6) The time-honoured mnemonic for immediate action is:
  A Airway maintenance with cervical spine control.
  B Breathing and ventilation.

C   Circulation with haemorrhage control.
D   Disability: brief neurological evaluation.
E   Exposure/environmental control: completely undress the patient, but prevent hypothermia.

IMMEDIATE MANAGEMENT

(1) *Airway*:
  (i)   Clear the airway by sucking out any debris, remove loose or broken dentures and insert an oropharyngeal airway. Give 100% oxygen by tight-fitting mask with reservoir bag. Aim for an oxygen saturation above 94%.
  (ii) Intubation:
    (a) If the gag reflex is absent or reduced, the patient requires intubating, ideally by a skilled doctor, e.g. an anaesthetist.
    (b) Take great care to minimise neck movements in the unconscious head injury or suspected neck injury by in-line manual immobilisation.
    (c) Use capnography to measure the end tidal CO_2 to confirm correct endotracheal tube placement.
  (iii) Cricothyrotomy: if intubation is impossible due to direct laryngeal injury or severe maxillofacial injury, proceed directly to cricothyrotomy (see page 31).
(2) *Maintain the integrity of the cervical spine*:
  (i)   Place the unconscious head injury and the suspected neck injury in a semi-rigid collar.
  (ii) Head movements must be minimised. When the patient requires turning, the body should be 'log rolled', holding the head in the neutral position at all times.
(3) *Breathing and ventilation*:
  (i)   Close a sucking chest wound with open pneumothorax using an occlusive dressing such as paraffin gauze under an adhesive film dressing (OpSite), secured along three sides only, leaving the fourth open for air to escape.

        (a) Proceed to formal intercostal tube drainage (see page 24).

  (ii) Tension pneumothorax:

        (a) Suspect a tension pneumothorax if the trachea is displaced away, with distended neck veins, unequal chest expansion and absent or decreased breath sounds.

        (b) Insert a wide-bore needle or cannula into the second intercostal space in the mid-clavicular line. If this is followed by the rush of released air, proceed to formal intercostal tube drainage (see page 24).

  (iii) Flail chest:

        (a) This will cause paradoxical movement of a part of the chest wall and may necessitate positive pressure ventilation.

        (b) An associated haemothorax or pneumothorax will require an intercostal tube drain to prevent the development of a tension pneumothorax when positive pressure ventilation is used.

(4) *Circulation with haemorrhage control*:

  (i) Apply a bulky sterile dressing to compress any external bleeding point (not a tourniquet, as this increases bleeding by venous congestion).

  (ii) Establish an intravenous infusion:

        (a) Insert two large-bore (14-gauge or 16-gauge) cannulae into the antecubital veins.

        (b) In mediastinal or neck injuries, one cannula should be below the diaphragm, e.g. in the femoral vein.

  (iii) Monitor the pulse, blood pressure, ECG and pulse oximetry.

  (iv) Take blood for haemoglobin, U&E, blood sugar and cross-match at least 4 units of blood according to the suspected injuries. Save serum for a drug screen in case alcohol or drug intoxication is subsequently suspected. Send arterial blood gases.

  (v) Infusion fluid:

(a) Infuse normal saline or a plasma expander such as polygeline (Haemaccel) to correct hypovolaemia.

(b) Remember in healthy adults loss of up to 30% of the blood volume, e.g. 1.5 litres, causes tachycardia with a narrowed pulse pressure only. Therefore, a consistent fall in systolic blood pressure indicates that at least 30% of the blood volume has already been lost.

(c) Change to blood if 1.5 litres of normal saline and 1 litre of Haemaccel fail to reverse the hypovolaemia. A full cross-match takes 1.5 h, type-specific cross-match 10 min and O rhesus-negative blood is available immediately.

(d) Use a blood warmer and macropore blood filter for multiple transfusions. Fresh frozen plasma 5 units and platelets may be required after transfusing 10 units of blood. Discuss this with the haematologist.

(vi) Cardiac tamponade:

(a) If there is persistent hypotension with distended neck veins that fill on inspiration (Kussmaul's sign), consider cardiac tamponade.

(b) Perform pericardiocentesis (see page 10) and call the surgical team for a decision on urgent thoracotomy.

(vii) A CVP line is useful, but should only be inserted by a skilled operator to avoid inadvertent arterial puncture or causing a pneumothorax.

(5) *Disability: brief neurological evaluation.*

(i) Assess the level of consciousness using the Glasgow Coma Scale (see page 128).

(ii) Examine the pupil size, pupil reactions and eye movements.

(iii) Assess for abnormal tone, weakness and gross sensory loss, or an asymmetric response to pain if the patient is unconscious. Check the limb reflexes including the plantar responses.

(iv) Examine the face and scalp for injuries (see page 141).

(6) *Exposure: completely undress the patient.*

    (i) Request a lateral cervical spine x-ray, CXR and pelvic x-ray.

    (ii) These are performed in the resuscitation bay without interrupting patient care.

(7) (i) Cover any exposed abdominal viscera with saline-soaked packs.

    (ii) Examine the front of the abdomen, including the perineum, for evidence of penetrating trauma or blunt trauma, e.g. the imprint of clothing or a tyre mark on the skin. Consider peritoneal lavage (see page 159).

    (iii) Examine the back for evidence of penetrating or blunt trauma. Palpate the spine for deformity and widened interspinous gaps.

(8) Assess the pelvis by springing to detect instability from major pelvic ring fracture, although this is an unreliable sign. Look for associated urethral injury.

    (i) Perform a rectal examination to assess the position of the prostate, integrity of the rectal wall, anal sphincter tone and to check for evidence of internal bleeding.

    (ii) If there is any bleeding from the urethral meatus, a scrotal haematoma or a high-riding prostate suspect urethral transection. Do not attempt urethral catheterisation.

    (iii) Otherwise, insert a urethral catheter and measure the urine output which should be over 50 ml/h in the adult, and 1 ml/kg per hour in a child.

(9) Pass a large-bore nasogastric tube, or orogastric tube if a basal skull or midface fracture are present. This is particularly important in children who commonly develop acute gastric dilatation following trauma.

(10) Splint major limb fractures, cover compound injuries with sterile dressings and check the peripheral pulses.

The above procedures will save life and allow a decision on priorities in proceeding to definitive care. Make sure an ongoing record is kept of all clinical findings and vital signs and keep re-examining the patient regularly. Obtain as full a history as possible from ambulance crew, witnesses or relatives as well as the patient. A useful mnemonic for the history is AMPLE:

A   Allergies;
M   Medications;
P   Past history, including alcohol and cigarette use;
L   Last meal;
E   Events/environment relating to the injury, including time, speed of impact, initial vital signs and any change in condition.

FURTHER DIAGNOSIS AND MANAGEMENT OF MULTIPLE INJURIES: DEFINITIVE CARE

This is considered under the following headings:

(1) Head and facial injuries:
  (i)   scalp;
  (ii)   face;
  (iii) eyes;
  (iv)   nose;
  (v)   mouth;
  (vi)   ears.

(2) Neck injuries:
  (i)   cervical spine injury;
  (ii)   neck sprain;
  (iii) airway injury;
  (iv)   vascular injury;
  (v)   nerve injury;
  (vi)   oesophageal injury.

(3) Chest injuries:
  (i)   pneumothorax;
  (ii)   haemothorax;
  (iii)   rib and sternum fractures;
  (iv)   myocardial contusion;
  (v)   aortic rupture;
  (vi)   diaphragm rupture;
  (vii)   oesophageal rupture;
  (viii) penetrating chest injuries.

(4) Abdominal injuries:
    (i)   penetrating injury;
    (ii)   blunt abdominal trauma.
(5) Pelvic and urethral injuries:
    (i)   pelvic injury;
    (ii)   bladder and urethral injury.
(6) Back injuries:
    (i)   thoracic and lumbar spine injury;
    (ii)   nonpenetrating renal injuries;
    (iii)   penetrating renal injuries.
(7) Limb injuries.

HEAD AND FACIAL INJURIES

(1) *Scalp.*
    (i)   Look for lacerations, haematomas, penetrating wounds, foreign bodies and palpate for evidence of deformity and fracture.
    (ii)   If a major head injury is suspected, assess the level of consciousness and manage as described on page 126.

(2) *Face.*
    (i)   Check the integrity of the airway again and remember the possibility of an unsuspected neck injury.
    (ii)   Look for bruising, swelling or deformity suggesting orbital, nasal, malar or mandibular fractures (see pages 334–8).
    (iii)   Look for parotid and facial nerve damage in injuries to the face in the area in front of the ear.
    (iv)   Clean and inspect all the facial lacerations. They will require meticulous debridement and suture when the patient's condition is stable and all serious injuries have been dealt with.

(3) *Eyes.*
    (i)   Inspect the eyes for evidence of penetrating or blunt injury, looking for iris prolapse, hyphaema and traumatic mydriasis (see page 318).
    (ii)   Check the visual acuity and eye movements.
    (iii)   Assess the pupil size and reactions and examine the fundi for evidence of vitreous or retinal haemorrhage and retinal detachment.

(4) *Nose*.
  (i)   Examine for evidence of blood or CSF leakage suggesting a basal skull fracture (see page 130).
  (ii) Palpate for deformity and nasal bone fracture (see page 302).
  (iii) Look specifically for a septal haematoma that will require incision and drainage if it is large, to reduce the risk of subsequent cartilage necrosis (see page 302).

(5) *Mouth*.
  (i)   Examine for broken or missing teeth. They may have been inhaled (see page 333).
  (ii) Check for dental malocclusion suggesting maxillary or mandibular fracture (see page 334).
  (iii) Assess for nasopharyngeal bleeding, which may be profuse and associated with a basal skull fracture. Look for any tongue lacerations, although they rarely need repairing (see page 332).

(6) *Ears*.
  (i)   Examine for skin and cartilage damage that will require drainage and suture later.
  (ii) Consider perforation of the eardrum, although if frank bleeding is seen, do not examine with a speculum to avoid introducing infection. This bleeding will be associated with a basal skull fracture or damage to the external ear canal (see page 298).

NECK INJURIES: CERVICAL SPINE INJURY

This should be considered in all patients with localised neck pain or stiffness following trauma. It should also be assumed in any unconscious head injury, and suspected in any multiply injured patient.

DIAGNOSIS

(1) If the patient is conscious ask about local pain, tenderness on palpation and associated limb weakness or sensory deficit.

(2) Palpate for areas of tenderness, swelling or deformity in the neck. Assess for limb tone, weakness, reflex loss and sensory deficit including loss of saddle area sensation and anal tone.

(3) A cervical or high thoracic cord lesion will cause respiratory difficulty, abdominal breathing and tachypnoea. Loss of sympathetic tone will cause bradycardia, hypotension and hypothermia from vasodilatation if the ambient temperature is low.

(4) Motor weakness should be described by myotome and reflex abnormalities:

    (i)   Myotomes in the upper limb:

Root	Action
C5	Shoulder abduction
C6, C7	Shoulder adduction
C5, C6	Elbow flexion
C7	Elbow extension
C6	Pronation and supination
(C6), C7	Wrist flexion
C6, (C7)	Wrist extension
C8	Finger flexion
C7	Finger extension
T1	Intrinsic hand muscles

    (ii)   Use the Medical Research Council scale to grade muscle weakness:

Grade 0	Complete paralysis
Grade 1	A flicker of contraction only
Grade 2	Movement only possible if gravity is eliminated
Grade 3	Movement against gravity
Grade 4	Movement against gravity and resistance
Grade 5	Normal power

    (iii)   Reflexes in the upper limb:

Root	Reflex
C5, (C6)	Biceps
(C5), C6	Supinator
(C6), C7, C8	Triceps

Use reinforcement (the Jendrassik manoeuvre) before concluding that a reflex is absent, e.g. ask the patient to clench the teeth hard or hold the knees together.

(5) Assess sensation by testing pain fibres using pinprick (spinothalamic tracts), and examine fine touch or joint position sense (posterior columns). Describe any changes by dermatome abnormalities:

    (i)   Dermatomes in the upper limb:

Root	Distribution
C5	Outer, upper arm
C6	Outer forearm
C7	Middle finger
C8	Inner forearm
T1	Inner, upper arm

    (ii)   C4 and T2 dermatomes are adjacent on the front of the chest at the level of the first and second ribs (C5 to T1 supply the upper limb).

(6) The myotomes, reflexes and dermatomes in the leg are described on page 259.

MANAGEMENT

(1) Always apply a semi-rigid collar in any suspected neck injury, minimise head movements and use laterally placed sandbags taped to the forehead to prevent head rotation.

(2) Urgent airway control with orotracheal or nasotracheal intubation may be required for hypoventilation. Ideally a skilled operator should perform this.

(3) Restore the circulatory volume if the patient is hypotensive. Look for sources of blood loss first, before deciding that the hypotension is due to vasodilatation with bradycardia from loss of sympathetic tone in a cervical cord injury (neurogenic shock).

(4) X-ray the neck:

    (i)   Lateral cervical spine: make sure all 7 cervical vertebrae and the C7/T1 junction are seen. Look for signs of displacement, wedge fracture, teardrop fracture, odontoid peg fracture and an increase in the soft-tissue shadow in front of the vertebral bodies (see Fig. 5).

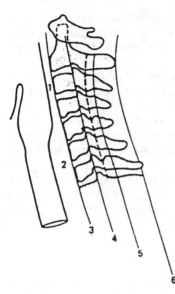

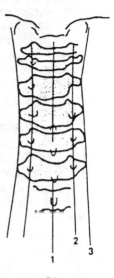

(a)   (b)

Fig. 5.
(a) Lateral cervical spine x-ray in the adult.
   1   Retropharyngeal space (less than 4 mm)
   2   Retrotracheal space (less than the width of one vertebral body)
   3   Anterior longitudinal ligament line
   4   Posterior longitudinal ligament line
   5   Spinolaminar line
   6   Posterior spinal line
   Lines 3–6 should all be parallel, following the normal gentle lordotic curve of the cervical spine. The spinal cord runs between lines 4 and 5.
(b) Anteroposterior cervical spine x-ray
   1   Interspinous line
   2   Foramen transversarium line
   3   Transverse processes line
   Lines 1–3 should be straight in the normal neck.

(a) The retropharyngeal space should be less than 4 mm at the level of C3.

(b) The retrotracheal space should be less than the width of one vertebral body in adults.

    (ii)   Open-mouth view for odontoid peg fracture.

    (iii)   Anteroposterior view: look for rotation of the vertebrae, loss of joint space and transverse process fracture.

(5) However, severe ligamentous damage may occur, leaving the neck unstable, with an apparently normal x-ray.

    (i)   This is more likely in children, in whom 50% of serious spinal injuries have normal x-rays (SCIWORA — spinal cord injury without radiological abnormality).

    (ii)   In elderly patients with cervical spondylosis, neck hyperextension may cause predominant weakness of the arms without any associated fracture or dislocation (central cord syndrome).

(6) Refer all suspected cervical spine injuries to the orthopaedic or surgical team and begin pressure area nursing.

(7) The use of high-dose methylprednisolone to improve neurological outcome in patients with complete or incomplete spinal cord damage is controversial:

    (i)   Infuse methylprednisolone 30 mg/kg over 15 min, followed 45 min later by 5.4 mg/kg per hour for 23 h.

    (ii)   Start treatment within 8 h of injury, guided by the advice of the regional Spinal Injuries Unit.

NECK INJURIES: NECK SPRAIN

DIAGNOSIS

(1) Hyperextension injury due to sudden deceleration in a motor vehicle accident is commonly termed whiplash injury.

    (i)   In practice, neck sprain occurs with other directions of impact including hyperflexion.

    (ii)   All result in neck pain and stiffness that typically occur 12–24 h after the injury, sometimes associated with headache.

(2) The pain may radiate to the shoulders and arms causing paraesthesiae, but neurological examination does not show any objective deficit.

(3) Neck movements are restricted by pain.

(4) Unfortunately symptoms may continue for months and be exacerbated by further minor injuries.

MANAGEMENT

(1) Request a cervical spine x-ray, which may show loss of the normal anterior curvature due to muscle spasm.

(2) Treat with a soft cervical collar and a nonsteroidal anti-inflammatory analgesic such as diclofenac 50 mg orally t.d.s.

(3) If the pain fails to settle, refer the patient to the physiotherapy department for early mobilisation exercises and heat treatment etc.

(4) Refer the patient to the orthopaedic clinic in the event the above measures are unsuccessful.

NECK INJURIES: AIRWAY INJURY

DIAGNOSIS

(1) Airway injuries may be penetrating or blunt, isolated or associated with multiple injury.

(2) They cause stridor, hoarseness, cough, haemoptysis and pain, with the development of local swelling, subcutaneous emphysema, pneumothorax or haemothorax.

(3) An anteroposterior and lateral cervical spine x-ray and CXR should be performed. The patient must never be left unattended at any stage.

MANAGEMENT

(1) Perform endotracheal intubation, cricothyrotomy or insert an endotracheal tube directly into a gaping wound in the trachea to maintain patency of the airway.

(2) Refer the patient immediately to the surgical team for admission.

NECK INJURIES: VASCULAR INJURY

DIAGNOSIS AND MANAGEMENT

(1) Vascular injury causes obvious external haemorrhage or internal bleeding, with rapid haematoma formation which may compromise the airway.

(2) (i) Do not attempt to probe or explore any penetrating wounds in the accident department. Leave all penetrating objects *in situ*.

   (ii) Refer the patient immediately to the surgical team for admission. The patient will require angiography and urgent surgical exploration in theatre.

NECK INJURIES: NERVE INJURY

DIAGNOSIS AND MANAGEMENT

(1) (i) Recurrent laryngeal branch of the vagus: damage to this nerve causes hoarseness and vocal cord paralysis.

   (ii) Accessory nerve damage causes loss of function of trapezius and sternomastoid.

   (iii) Phrenic nerve damage causes loss of diaphragmatic movement.

   (iv) Hypoglossal nerve damage causes deviation of the tongue to the affected side.

   (v) Cervical sympathetic cord damage causes Horner's syndrome with partial ptosis, a constricted pupil and decreased sweating on the same side of the face.

(2) Refer all these injuries to the surgical team.

NECK INJURIES: OESOPHAGEAL INJURY

DIAGNOSIS AND MANAGEMENT

(1) Oesophageal injury causes dysphagia, drooling and localised pain with the development of surgical emphysema.

(2) Refer this rare condition to the surgical team for immediate admission.

PNEUMOTHORAX

DIAGNOSIS

(1) Tension pneumothorax:
- (i)   This causes severe respiratory distress, tachypnoea and hypotension. There is tracheal deviation away from the affected side, distended neck veins, loss of chest expansion on the affected side, a hyperresonant percussion note and diminished or absent breath sounds.
- (ii) It requires immediate decompression. Use a large-bore intravenous cannula inserted into the second intercostal space in the mid-clavicular line, followed by the insertion of an intercostal drain (see page 24).

(2) Simple pneumothorax:
- (i)   This is surprisingly easy to miss; examine for decreased chest expansion, quiet breath sounds and subcutaneous emphysema.
- (ii) It is caused by blunt or penetrating chest trauma, and penetrating abdominal trauma breaching the diaphragm.
- (iii) An erect CXR, taken on expiration to highlight a small apical pneumothorax, confirms the diagnosis.
  - (a) A supine CXR may however appear normal and miss a small pneumothorax lying anteriorly.

MANAGEMENT

(1) This is by insertion of an intercostal drain into the fifth or sixth intercostal space in the midaxillary line (see page 24).
(2) Virtually all cases of traumatic pneumothorax require a chest drain to avoid the subsequent development of tension, especially if positive pressure ventilation is necessary.

HAEMOTHORAX

DIAGNOSIS

(1) This results from chest wall damage, penetrating or blunt lung injury and great vessel damage.
(2) It causes hypotension, respiratory difficulty with reduced chest expansion, quiet breath sounds and a dull percussion note at the base of the lung.
(3) An erect or semi-erect chest x-ray is necessary to identify a fluid level.
(4) If only a supine CXR is possible, assess for evidence of diffuse haziness over one hemithorax, which is easily overlooked. Alternatively a lateral decubitus CXR may be taken.

MANAGEMENT

(1) Give high-dose oxygen and commence intravenous fluid replacement.
(2) Insert a large-bore 32 or 36 French gauge intercostal drain in the fifth or sixth intercostal space in the midaxillary line, using blunt dissection down to and through the pleura (see page 24).
(3) Autotransfusion devices are available to collect and return the intrathoracic blood to the circulation, providing contamination from gastrointestinal injury is excluded.
(4) Otherwise, if bleeding is severe and persists, a thoracotomy may be required (see page 156).

CHEST INJURIES: RIB AND STERNUM FRACTURES

DIAGNOSIS

(1) These cause localised pain and tenderness, worse on breathing or springing the chest wall, following direct trauma.

(2) A CXR is indicated to look for the complications of a pneumothorax, haemothorax and a widened mediastinum, not simply to visualise the fractures.

(3) A lateral sternal x-ray is indicated for a suspected sternal fracture, and an ECG to exclude myocardial contusion (see page 152).

(4) Associated injury may occur with fractures in the following areas:

    (i) *Clavicle, first and second ribs*: damage to the subclavian vessels, aorta, trachea, main bronchus and spinal cord or brachial plexus.

    (ii) *Sternum*: damage to the myocardium, great vessels and upper thoracic spine.

    (iii) *Right lower ribs*: damage to the liver and right kidney.

    (iv) *Left lower ribs*: damage to the spleen and left kidney.

MANAGEMENT

(1) A flail segment with paradoxical chest wall movement from multiple rib fractures in two sites, causes hypoxia mainly from underlying pulmonary contusion.

    (i) Give the patient oxygen, check the blood gases and refer to the surgical team for pain relief possibly by thoracic epidural.

    (ii) Positive pressure ventilation may be required for deteriorating respiratory function, after insertion of an intercostal drain for any pneumothorax, however small.

(2) Refer the following patients to the surgical team for admission after resuscitation, insertion of an intercostal drain if indicated and adequate analgesia such as diclofenac 75 mg i.m.

    (i) Pneumothorax, haemothorax;

    (ii) Fractured sternum with severe pain or ECG abnormalities;

    (iii) Complications in (4) (i) to (iv) above;

    (iv) Pre-existing lung disease with poor respiratory reserve;

    (v)   Rib fractures with significant pain.
(3) The remaining patients with uncomplicated rib fractures or an isolated sternal fracture with a normal ECG and CXR may be discharged:
    (i)   Provide an analgesic such as paracetamol 500 mg and codeine phosphate 8 mg (co-codamol) two tablets orally q.d.s.;
    (ii)   Recommend regular deep breathing exercises to prevent atelectasis;
    (iii) Contact the general practitioner by telephone or letter.

MYOCARDIAL CONTUSION

DIAGNOSIS

(1) This is due to blunt deceleration injury and is associated with rib fractures, sternal fracture and chest wall contusion. It is difficult to diagnose.
(2) It may be asymptomatic, cause chest pain or rarely transient right ventricular dysfunction with distended neck veins and hypotension.
(3) ECG abnormalities range from sinus tachycardia, atrial fibrillation, bundle branch block and ventricular extrasystoles to nonspecific ST and T wave abnormalities or ST elevation.
(4) Cardiac enzyme changes including creatine phosphokinase (CK) and CK-MB isoenzymes are unreliable. They may however incidentally diagnose antecedent myocardial infarction.
(5) Echocardiography may show wall motion abnormalities, but is most useful to exclude cardiac tamponade or acute valvular rupture.

MANAGEMENT

(1) Give the patient high-dose oxygen and attach a cardiac monitor. Gain intravenous access, send blood for FBC, cardiac enzymes and G&S, and give a fluid challenge if there is hypotension.

(2) Consider morphine 2.5–5 mg i.v. with an antiemetic such as metoclopramide 10 mg i.v. for pain.

(3) Perform a 12-lead ECG and refer the patient for cardiac monitoring if there are any ECG abnormalities. Obtain an urgent echocardiogram if hypotension persists or cardiac tamponade cannot be excluded.

AORTIC RUPTURE

DIAGNOSIS

(1) This occurs from a high-speed deceleration injury when the aorta is torn just distal to the left subclavian artery.

(2) Only 10–15% of patients with rupture of the thoracic aorta survive to reach hospital. Always consider this diagnosis in any deceleration injury over 45 miles per hour or a fall from over 15 feet.

(3) Look for chest or interscapular pain, unequal blood pressure in each arm, or a different femoral and brachial pulse volume. In contained aortic rupture, initial hypotension will respond to modest fluid replacement.

(4) Perform a CXR to look for signs of aortic rupture:
  (i)   Widened mediastinum (8 cm or more in a 1-m supine AP x-ray).
     (a) about 10% of angiograms for a widened mediastinum will subsequently show contained aortic rupture;
     (b) other causes of a widened mediastinum include sternal fracture and lower cervical or thoracic spine fracture with mediastinal haematoma.[1]
  (ii) blurred aortic outline with obliteration of the aortic knuckle;
  (iii) left apical cap of fluid in the pleural space and a left haemothorax;
  (iv) depressed left main stem bronchus;
  (v)   displacement of the trachea to the right;
  (vi) displacement of a nasogastric tube in the oesophagus to the right.

MANAGEMENT

(1) Insert two large-bore intravenous cannulae, cross-match at least 10 units of blood and give fluid cautiously. Avoid overtransfusion or hypertension from poorly controlled pain etc.
(2) Look for a cervical, thoracic or sternal fracture clinically and by x-ray, although exclusion of aortic rupture is still necessary irrespective of these, if the CXR is suggestive.
(3) Refer the patient to the surgical team for aortography or transoesophageal echo, followed by urgent thoracotomy and repair if positive.

DIAPHRAGM RUPTURE

DIAGNOSIS

(1) This may occur from blunt or penetrating chest or abdominal trauma including crush fracture of the pelvis. It causes difficulty in breathing and occasionally bowel sounds are audible in the chest.
(2) Left-sided lesions are more common and allow eventration of the stomach or intestine into the chest.
(3) The diagnosis is often missed as the CXR appears normal in 25% of cases, although a haemothorax, pneumothorax, elevated hemidiaphragm and coils of bowel or a nasogastric tube curled up in the left lower chest may be seen.

MANAGEMENT

(1) Carefully insert an intercostal drain for any associated haemothorax or pneumothorax, using blunt dissection down to and through the parietal pleura (see page 24). Never use the trocar introducer to insert the drain.
(2) Decompress the stomach with a nasogastric tube.
(3) Refer the patient to the surgical team.

OESOPHAGEAL RUPTURE

DIAGNOSIS

(1) This rare injury is most commonly from penetrating trauma or blunt trauma from a blow to the upper abdomen. Other causes include instrumentation, swallowing a sharp object and spontaneous rupture from vomiting (Boerhaave's syndrome).
(2) There is retrosternal pain, difficulty in swallowing sometimes with haematemesis and subcutaneous emphysema.
(3) CXR shows a widened mediastinum with mediastinal air, a left pneumothorax, pleural effusion or haemothorax. These findings in the absence of rib fracture should suggest the possibility of rupture.

MANAGEMENT

(1) Give the patient oxygen, establish venous access with a large-bore intravenous cannula and replace fluids. Give morphine 2.5–5 mg i.v. for pain with an antiemetic.
(2) Carefully insert an intercostal drain. Particulate matter in the intercostal tube drainage would confirm the diagnosis.
(3) If rupture is considered likely, commence broad-spectrum antibiotics such as ampicillin 1 g i.v., gentamicin 80 mg i.v. and metronidazole 500 mg i.v.
(4) Refer the patient to the surgical team for a gastrografin swallow and/or oesophagoscopy, followed by surgical repair if feasible.

PENETRATING CHEST INJURIES

DIAGNOSIS

(1) These injuries present with difficulty in breathing due to pain, pneumothorax, haemothorax or tension pneumothorax. However, some patients are surprisingly undistressed.

(2) Hypotension occurs due to blood loss, cardiac tamponade or the development of tension.

(3) A CXR may show some of the above complications,
although airway management, needle thoracocentesis and
fluid resuscitation must be performed first when indicated.

(4) Remember that penetrating wounds:

   (i)   Medial to the nipple-line or tips of the scapulae
         posteriorly are at high risk of heart or great vessel
         injury;

   (ii) Below the fourth intercostal space may also injure
         the abdominal contents;

   (iii) Above the umbilicus may injure the lungs, heart
         or great vessels.

MANAGEMENT

(1) Eighty per cent of penetrating chest injuries are
managed conservatively by insertion of an intercostal
drain (see page 24).

(2) Injuries involving the heart and great vessels will require
thoracotomy.

   (i)   *Indications for immediate emergency department
         thoracotomy:*[4]

         (a) Traumatic cardiac arrest, or near cardiac
             arrest, with vital signs (palpable pulse and
             spontaneous respirations) observed at the
             scene of the accident and a short prehospital
             transit time (up to 10 min, particularly when
             intubated).

         (b) Cardiac arrest from penetrating thoracic
             trauma due to a stab wound or a low-velocity
             bullet, as opposed to blunt chest trauma or a
             high-velocity bullet. The latter two are virtu-
             ally always fatal if cardiac arrest occurs.

         (c) Absence of major brain injury.

   (ii) *Indications for urgent elective thoracotomy:*

         (a) Cardiac tamponade following trauma that
             recurs after pericardiocentesis.

         (b) Massive haemothorax with greater than 1500
             ml initial drainage or over 200 ml/h for 4 h.

    (c) Penetrating cardiac injuries.

    (d) Persistent large air leak suggesting tracheo-bronchial injury.

PENETRATING ABDOMINAL INJURIES

DIAGNOSIS

(1) An entry wound may be obvious, with evisceration of bowel, or may be difficult to find if it is hidden by a gluteal fold or in the perineum.

(2) Associated damage to the chest can occur with any wound above the umbilicus.

(3) The most important signs to look for are hypotension and shock. Local rigidity and guarding with reduced bowel sounds occur but are less common.

(4) The causes include:

    (i)   Stabbing with a knife or hand-held sharp instrument.

    (ii) Industrial accidents, road accidents and explosions.

    (iii) Gunshot wounds. These may be divided into three types:

        (a) *High-velocity wound.* The muzzle velocity of a bullet from a high-velocity rifle exceeds 1000 m/s and a small entry wound is associated with gross internal tissue damage from cavitation, and a large exit wound.

        (b) *Low-velocity wound.* The muzzle velocity from a handgun reaches 250 m/s and the bullet causes local internal damage by perforation and laceration, often passing through several structures.

        (c) *Shotgun wound.* This causes massive superficial internal damage from close range (less than 7 m) and is usually fatal from a range of less than 3 m.

           If the shotgun is fired from more than 7 m, there is scattering of shot, perforating structures within the abdomen. A shot from over 40 m may not even penetrate the peritoneal cavity.

MANAGEMENT

(1) Cover any exposed bowel with saline-soaked pads.
(2) Give oxygen, send blood for FBC, cross-match, U&E, and amylase, and replace fluid initially with normal saline.
(3) Commence broad-spectrum antibiotics, e.g. ampicillin 1 g i.v., gentamicin 80 mg i.v. and metronidazole 500 mg i.v. Give tetanus prophylaxis.
(4) Request a CXR to look for associated thoracic injury. An abdominal x-ray is indicated to assess for metallic foreign bodies.
(5) Test the urine for blood indicating a urological injury although it is an unreliable sign.
(6) Refer all patients to the surgical team for urgent admission and laparotomy for all gunshot wounds and the majority of stab wounds.

BLUNT ABDOMINAL TRAUMA

DIAGNOSIS

(1) This should be suspected following a road traffic accident or a fall from a height, particularly if there is evidence of chest, pelvic or long-bone injury (e.g. injuries on either side of the abdomen).
  (i)   It should also be suspected when there is unexplained hypotension in the absence of obvious external bleeding or a thoracic injury.
(2) Look for the imprint of clothing or tyre marks as indicators of potential blunt abdominal injury. Bruising from a seat belt may overlie duodenal, pancreatic or small bowel injury and fracture-dislocation of the lumbar spine.
(3) Ask about referred shoulder-tip pain or localised pain suggesting lower rib, pelvic or thoracolumbar spine injury.
(4) Examine the chest, pelvis and back as well as the abdomen. Inspect the perineum and perform a rectal examination and a vaginal examination in the female.

(5) X-ray: an erect CXR, pelvic x-ray and lumbosacral spine x-ray are of more benefit than a plain abdominal film.

    (i)   Erect CXR: this may demonstrate a thoracic injury or free gas under the diaphragm. Look particularly for lower rib fractures associated with liver, splenic and renal injury.

    (ii)   Pelvic x-ray: a fractured pelvis may be associated with major abdominal injuries and must always be excluded.

    (iii) Plain abdominal film: look for loss of the psoas shadow, transverse process fracture, abnormal renal outlines and free gas within the peritoneal cavity on a lateral decubitus view.

MANAGEMENT

(1) Give oxygen and send blood for FBC, U&E, blood sugar, amylase and cross-match at least 4 units of whole blood.

(2) Insert a large-bore intravenous cannula. Transfuse initially with crystalloid (e.g. normal saline) or colloid (e.g. polygeline – Haemaccel), then whole blood when available.

(3) Insert a urethral catheter to measure the urine output and to look for haematuria.

    (i)   Omit this if a urethral injury is suspected from blood at the meatus, a scrotal haematoma or a high-riding prostate on rectal examination.

    (ii)   Pass a nasogastric tube to drain the stomach.

(4) Indications for immediate laparotomy include:

    (i)   Persistent shock;

    (ii)   Rigid, silent abdomen;

    (iii) Radiological evidence of free gas or ruptured diaphragm.

(5) If immediate laparotomy is not indicated, consider diagnostic peritoneal lavage (DPL):

    (i)   DPL is used for unexplained hypotension in suspected abdominal injury or when abdominal examination is:

        (a) unreliable due to coma, intoxication or spinal injury;

      (b) equivocal due to fractured lower ribs, pelvis or lumbar spine;

      (c) impractical in planned extra-abdominal radiographic or surgical procedures.

(ii)   Insert a nasogastric and urethral catheter first.

(iii)   Perform the lavage by a mini-laparotomy technique using local anaesthetic with adrenaline then open dissection through all the layers of the abdominal wall.

(iv)   The admitting surgical team should perform the procedure which is positive if:

      (a) more than 10 ml of frank blood or enteric contents are aspirated;

      (b) peritoneal lavage fluid effluent exits via a chest tube or bladder catheter;

      (c) laboratory analysis of lavage fluid shows over 100 000 red blood cells/mm^3.

(v)   It is highly sensitive for intraperitoneal bleeding, but does not rule out retroperitoneal injury to the duodenum, pancreas, kidney and pelvis or diaphragm rupture.

(6) Alternatively, abdominal ultrasound may be used to look for free intraperitoneal fluid or evidence of parenchymal damage. It is rapid, repeatable, as sensitive as DPL and may also be performed at the bedside.

(7) CT scan should only be done if the patient is haemodynamically stable. It provides anatomical details including the retroperitoneum and may allow nonoperative management of some injuries.

PELVIC INJURIES

The major complication of a pelvic fracture is blood loss that may be massive, with up to 3 litres or more of concealed haemorrhage that may continue despite resuscitation.

DIAGNOSIS

(1) Pelvic injuries may result from direct trauma in road, work or sports accidents, and from falls.

(2) There is local pain, tenderness and bruising. Bony instability is demonstrated by distracting the iliac crests,
although this an unreliable sign.

(3) Associated bladder, urethral, vaginal and rectal
injuries occur which account for further morbidity. A
ruptured diaphragm must also be excluded (see page
154).

(4) Pelvic x-ray should always be performed in all multiple
injury patients especially if there is unexplained
hypotension. Pelvic fractures associated with the greatest risk of haemorrhage include:
  (i)   Straddle fracture of all 4 pubic rami;
  (ii) Open-book fracture with diastasis of the symph-
        ysis pubis over 2.5 cm;
  (iii) Vertical shear fracture.

MANAGEMENT

(1) Give oxygen, send blood for FBC, U&E and blood
sugar, cross-match at least 6 units of blood, and
commence an intravenous infusion.

(2) Do not attempt to catheterise the bladder if urethral
rupture is suspected, but await experienced surgical
assistance.

(3) Refer the patient immediately to the orthopaedic team.
External fixation of fractures, arterial embolisation and
laparotomy may be required for severe bleeding or a
urological injury.

(4) If hypotension persists, consider the temporary use of a
pneumatic antishock garment such as MAST (military
antishock trousers):
  (i)   These have three independent compartments,
        reducing the circulation through the pelvis and
        legs, thus supporting the blood pressure and
        splinting any fractures;
  (ii) The garment must never be deflated until rapid
        fluid replacement therapy and immediate laparo-
        tomy are available.

BLADDER AND URETHRAL INJURIES

DIAGNOSIS

(1) These injuries may occur particularly with major pelvic fractures or from a direct blow to the lower abdomen.

(2) *Bladder rupture*: this occurs intraperitoneally causing shock and peritonism, or extraperitoneally causing urine extravasation, local bruising and frank haematuria.

(3) *Urethral rupture*:
  (i) Membranous urethra.
     (a) Membranous urethral rupture causes difficulty voiding urine and urethral bleeding, which mimics extraperitoneal rupture of the bladder.
     (b) Rectal examination reveals a high-riding prostate, often with an underlying boggy haematoma.
  (ii) Bulbous urethra. Bulbous urethral rupture is caused by a fall astride an object resulting in local perineal bruising, pain and bleeding.

MANAGEMENT

(1) Do not attempt to catheterise the patient with a bladder or urethral injury.

(2) Treat the patient for pain and shock and give antibiotics such as ampicillin 1 g i.v. and gentamicin 80 mg i.v.

(3) Refer to the surgical team for an intravenous urogram, cystogram or ascending urethrogram as indicated.

BACK INJURIES

Always examine the back in multiple injury patients, carefully log-rolling patients with suspected spinal injury.

THORACIC AND LUMBAR SPINE INJURY

DIAGNOSIS

(1) This type of injury is caused by blunt trauma from a fall, a direct blow or in a traffic accident. A fractured

sternum may accompany a hyperflexion wedge fracture of the upper thoracic spine.

(2) Look for bruising, deformity and evidence of any penetrating injury.

(3) Palpate for localised tenderness and swelling around the vertebral column or an abnormal gap between the spinous processes suggesting a fracture, or overlying the renal areas suggesting a kidney injury (see page 164).

(4) Perform a careful neurological examination assessing for sensory deficit and a sensory level, loss of perianal sensation, and for motor and reflex loss in the legs (see page 259).

(5) The spinal cord ends at the level of the first lumbar vertebra, so any injury distal to this involves the cauda equina only.

(6) Thoracolumbar spine x-rays are indicated in the following high-risk patients:[5]

  (i)   Fall from 10 feet (3 metres);
  (ii)   High speed accident over 50 mph (80 kph);
  (iii) Ejection from motor vehicle or motor cycle;
  (iv)   GCS score 8 or less;
  (v)   Neurological deficit;
  (vi)   Back pain or tenderness (may be absent).

(7) These x-rays may show a wedge fracture, dislocation (particularly between T12 and L1, and L4 and L5) or a transverse process fracture.

MANAGEMENT

(1) Treat associated thoracic and abdominal injuries as a priority, log rolling the patient and minimising unneces sary movements, as thoracolumbar fractures are commonly unstable.

(2) Commence intravenous fluids and send blood for FBC, U&E, blood sugar and cross-match if there is hypotension from local or retroperitoneal bleeding or loss of sympathetic tone in high thoracic cord injury.

(3) Refer the patient to the orthopaedic team.

NONPENETRATING RENAL INJURIES

These may be associated with injury to the vertebral column, lower ribs, ureters, aorta, inferior vena cava and the abdominal contents.

DIAGNOSIS

(1) Loin pain and tenderness occur, which in association with haematuria suggest renal trauma.
(2) Hypotension is due to retroperitoneal bleeding or an associated paralytic ileus. A flank mass may be felt.
(3) Request a plain abdominal film and look for 11th and 12th rib fractures, loss of the psoas shadow or an abnormal soft-tissue outline indicating retroperitoneal bleeding.
(4) Intravenous urography is performed for suspected renal injury, although ultrasound or CT scanning may be preferred. Indications for radiology of the kidney and ureters include:
   (i) Macroscopic haematuria;
   (ii) Microscopic haematuria with shock (systolic BP 90 mmHg or less);
   (iii) Significant deceleration with the risk of renal pedicle injury;
   (iv) Local physical signs;
   (v) Penetrating proximity trauma (see below).

MANAGEMENT

(1) Resuscitate the patient with intravenous fluids and send blood for FBC, U&E, blood sugar and cross-match 2–6 units of blood.
(2) Consider peritoneal lavage to exclude associated intra-abdominal injuries.
(3) Refer the patient to the surgical team. Over 85 per cent of blunt renal injuries settle on conservative management with bed rest and analgesia.

PENETRATING RENAL INJURIES

These are rare and usually involve injury to the abdominal contents, ureter or vertebral column. They may be multiple or associated with penetrating injury at the front of the trunk.

DIAGNOSIS

(1) There is usually haematuria, localised pain and tenderness, although significant renal or ureteric injury may be present without haematuria.
(2) Ureteric colic may occur from the passage of blood clots.

MANAGEMENT

(1) Resuscitate the patient with intravenous fluids, and send blood for FBC, U&E and cross-match.
(2) Give tetanus prophylaxis as indicated.
(3) Refer the patient to the surgical team for intravenous urography. This will not only demonstrate the nature of the renal injury but also confirm the presence and normal function of the other kidney.

LIMB INJURIES

The management of limb injuries does not take precedence over head, thoracic, abdominal or pelvic injuries in the multiply injured patient, even though they may appear more dramatic and attract instant attention. Limb injuries are covered in detail in the Orthopaedic Section.

DIAGNOSIS

(1) Look for obvious deformity, swelling, tenderness, abnormal movement or crepitus (if the patient is unconscious).
(2) Check the distal pulses, particularly in a supracondylar humeral fracture or a dislocated knee.
(3) Remember that closed fractures bleed extensively with little external evidence, and open fractures bleed an even greater amount:

Site of closed fracture:	Predicted blood loss:
Pelvic ring	Up to 6 units or more
Femoral shaft	2–4 units
Tibial shaft	1–3 units

(4) Note any neurological deficit, e.g. radial nerve damage in a humeral shaft fracture or sciatic nerve damage in posterior hip dislocation.

MANAGEMENT

(1) Restore any deformity to a normal anatomical alignment. This is particularly important in a dislocated ankle, to prevent ischaemic pressure necrosis of the skin overlying the malleolus (see page 245).

(2) Cover compound fractures with a sterile dressing. Give flucloxacillin 1 g i.v. and benzylpenicillin 1 Mu (600 mg) i.v., and tetanus prophylaxis.

(3) Give increments of morphine 2.5–5 mg i.v. for severe pain with an antiemetic such as metoclopramide 10 mg i.v.

(4) Immobilise the fracture using a plaster of Paris backslab, or a specially designed splint such as the Donway traction splint for femoral shaft fractures.

    (i) Splinting reduces pain, making handling easier; it also reduces blood loss and the risk of neurovascular injury.

(5) Obtain urgent orthopaedic assistance if distal ischaemia is present. Otherwise refer the patient when the other major injuries have been stabilised.

(6) Traumatic amputation:

    (i) Control haemorrhage by direct pressure and elevation of the stump.

    (ii) Consider the possibility of replantation especially in a clean, sliced wound without crushing:

        (a) preserve the amputated part by wrapping in a sterile dressing soaked in saline;

        (b) seal the wrapped part in a sterile, dry plastic bag and immerse in a container of crushed ice and water;

        (c) give intravenous antibiotics and tetanus prophylaxis as for a compound fracture;

(d) x-ray the limb and severed part;
(e) refer the patient to the orthopaedic or plastic surgery team for consideration of microvascular surgery ideally performed within 6 h of injury.

BURNS

These are considered in the following categories:
 (1) Major burns;
 (2) Minor burns and scalds;
 (3) Electrocution and electrical burns;
 (4) Chemical burns;
 (5) Bitumen burns.

MAJOR BURNS

DIAGNOSIS

(1) History:
   (i) Ascertain the nature of the fire, how it started, whether there was any explosion, and how much delay there was in reaching hospital.
   (ii) Ask if the patient was in an enclosed place, if so for how long, and whether smoke or fumes were present which predispose to carbon monoxide and cyanide poisoning.
   (iii) Ask about previous respiratory or cardiac problems, present drug therapy, known allergies and tetanus status.
(2) Examine for signs of a respiratory burn:
   (i) Look for burns around the face and neck, burnt nasal hairs, and soot particles in the nose and mouth.
   (ii) Listen for signs of hoarseness, stridor or wheezing.
   (iii) Assess for headache and confusion suggesting carbon monoxide poisoning.
(3) Check for associated injuries and circulatory collapse.

(4) Determine the extent of the burn:
  (i)   In adults, use Wallace's 'rule of nines', ignoring areas of mere erythema (see Fig. 6).
  (ii) In children the head is relatively larger (12–14%) and the legs relatively smaller (14%), so use comparison with the size of the child's palm (equal to 1% of body surface area) when estimating the extent of the burn.

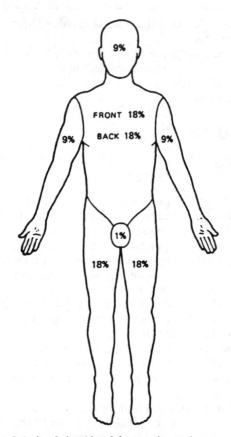

Fig. 6. Wallace's 'rule of nines' in adults to estimate the percentage body area burned.

(5) Determine the depth of the burn:
  (i)   *Full-thickness*. The skin is white or brown, dry, leathery, anaesthetic with no capillary refill. This will require skin grafting.
  (ii) *Partial-thickness*:
        (a) Deep dermal. The skin is pink or white, feels thickened, does not blanch and has reduced sensation. This should heal over in about 3 weeks, but some areas may require grafting to avoid leaving a scar.
        (b) Superficial. The skin is red and blistered, blanches and is painful. This should heal spontaneously in 10–14 days.
  (iii) *Superficial*. Erythema, blanching and pain occur, followed by peeling as in a sunburn. This should heal rapidly by 5–7 days.

MANAGEMENT

(1) For a respiratory burn and smoke inhalation:
  (i)   Check the adequacy of the airway, give 100% oxygen by tight-fitting mask with reservoir bag and nebulised salbutamol 5 mg for wheezing.
  (ii) Send blood for a carboxyhaemoglobin level which will confirm exposure to carbon monoxide (see page 76 for further management of carbon monoxide poisoning). Check the blood gases and monitor the ECG and pulse oximetry.
  (iii) Request a CXR.
  (iv) Call the anaesthetist immediately to pass a cuffed endotracheal tube for deep burns of the face, tongue and pharynx, stridor, hoarseness or a deteriorating level of consciousness.
  (v)   Consider the possibility of cyanide poisoning from burning plastics and fabrics,[6] especially in patients with tachypnoea, coma, convulsions, cardiac arrhythmias, hypotension and acidosis:
        (a) act immediately on circumstantial evidence of cyanide poisoning as no rapid measurement is available;

    (b) ventilate the patient with 100% oxygen;

    (c) in those seriously ill with coma and cardio-respiratory failure and if the diagnosis is highly likely, give 1.5% dicobalt edetate (Kelocyanor) 20 ml i.v. immediately over 1 min followed by 50% dextrose 50 ml i.v.;

    (d) repeat the dicobalt edetate if the response is inadequate, followed by a third dose after a further 5 min if necessary.

(2) Intravenous infusion:

    (i) Commence intravenous fluids in any burn over 10% in a child or 15% in an adult, or for associated injuries causing hypovolaemia.

    (ii) Insert a large-bore (14-gauge or 16-gauge) cannula using an antecubital fossa vein or cut-down technique. Avoid central line insertion as there is a high risk of sepsis from this procedure.

    (iii) Send blood for Hb, PCV, U&E, blood sugar, G&S and a drug screen if there is suspected alcohol or drug abuse.

    (iv) Give a volume of fluid according to the Muir and Barclay formula:

$$\frac{\text{Percentage area of burn x Weight (kg)}}{2}.$$

    (a) This amount of fluid in millilitres should be given in each of three time periods: 0–4 h, 4–8 h and 8–12 h from the time the burn was sustained.

    (b) Rapid fluid replacement may initially be required to catch up, if there has been a delay in reaching hospital.

    (v) Type of fluid:

    (a) The quantity of fluid is more important than the type. Use plasma protein fraction (PPF) or 5% human albumin solution as plasma expanders;

    (b) Give polygeline (Haemaccel) initially in extensive, deep (e.g. electrical) burns or when resuscitation is delayed as it promotes a solute diuresis;

(c) Alternatively, a crystalloid solution alone such as compound sodium lactate (Hartmann's) may be given but at the rate of 4 ml/kg per percentage body surface area burned, 50% in the first 8 h and 50% in the remaining 16 h.

(3) Insert a urinary catheter to assess the adequacy of transfusion, aiming for an hourly urine output of 50 ml in adults. Pass a nasogastric tube in patients with burns over 20%, who may develop gastric stasis.

(4) Analgesia and sedation:
  (i) Opiates. Give morphine 2.5–5 mg i.v. with an antiemetic such as metoclopramide 10 mg i.v.
  (ii) Trimeprazine syrup (Vallergan) is a useful sedative in children. Give an initial dose of 2 mg/kg.
  (iii) Remember undertransfusion or hypoxia are commoner causes of restlessness than pain.

(5) Give tetanus prophylaxis to all burn patients.

(6) Escharotomy:
  (i) Circumferential leathery, full-thickness burns may cause difficulty in breathing by constricting chest wall movements, and distal ischaemia in a limb or digits by restricting the blood flow.
  (ii) Request the surgical team to perform relieving incisions through the burn area. This is known as escharotomy, and does not require an anaesthetic.

(7) Wound dressing:
  (i) Leave any adherent clothing alone and do not break blisters in the burnt area.
  (ii) Cover the burn with a nonadherent, paraffin-impregnated gauze (Jelonet) dressing or saline soaked gauze pads. Beware causing hypothermia in children if too many wet soaks are used.
  (iii) Avoid silver sulphadiazine (Flamazine) cream until the patient has been fully assessed by the surgical or burns unit team.

(8) Admission:
  (i) All major burns will require hospital admission by the surgical team.

   (ii)   Refer patients to a specialist burns unit with:
          (a) burns over 10% in children and 15% in
               adults;
          (b) burns of important functional areas such as
               the face, hands and genitalia;
          (c) respiratory burns;
          (d) chemical burns and electrical burns including
               lightning injury.
   (iii) Serious burns must be fully assessed and resusci-
          tated before departure, similar to the precautions
          taken when transferring serious head injuries to a
          neurosurgical unit.
   (iv)   Avoid the risk of the patient developing sudden
          respiratory obstruction during transit, by prior
          endotracheal intubation of a significant respira-
          tory burn by an experienced anaesthetist.

Note: burn injuries are always frightening and unexpected,
and relatives (particularly parents of children) may initially
feel guilty and angry. Special counselling and reassurance is
needed from an early stage to help them come to terms with
the injuries and to allay their anxieties, so they may be a
useful support to the victim.

MINOR BURNS AND SCALDS

These include full-thickness burns under 1%, or partial-thickness burns under 15% body surface area in adults and under
10% in children. The aim is to manage them as outpatients, in
distinction from patients with major burns who require
admission (see above).

INITIAL MANAGEMENT

 (1) Irrigate the wound immediately with copious running
     cold water until the pain is relieved.
 (2) Assess the extent and depth of the burn (see page 168).
     (i)   In general, superficial partial-thickness burns heal
           spontaneously, deep dermal partial-thickness
           burns heal slowly with scar formation and full-

thickness burns do not heal at all, unless under 1–2 cm in diameter when epithelium will cover the area from the edges. Otherwise grafting is required.

(3) Clean with saline or an antiseptic, e.g. chlorhexidine.

(4) Give an analgesic such as codeine phosphate 30–60 mg orally for adults, or paracetamol elixir 120–250 mg for children.

(5) Deroof large blisters that have broken, or aspirate the fluid if the blister is tense. Otherwise leave blisters intact to protect the healing epithelium.

(6) Apply silver sulphadiazine cream (Flamazine) and cover the burn with a nonadherent paraffin-impregnated gauze dressing (Jelonet).

(7) Then apply gauze and an absorbent layer of cotton-wool or a Gamgee pad, overlapping the paraffin-impregnated gauze dressing by 3 cm either end.

(8) Finally keep the absorbent layer in place with a firm crêpe bandage, again overlapping each end by 3 cm, sealing with Elastoplast.

(9) Always elevate the limb using a high-arm sling for arm and hand burns.

(10) Give tetanus prophylaxis and analgesics to take home, such as codeine phosphate 30–60 mg orally q.d.s., or paracetamol 500 mg and codeine phosphate 8 mg (co-codamol) two tablets q.d.s.

(11) Remember that burns of the perineum, feet or hands in children may be due to nonaccidental injury. Suspect this when there has been a delay in seeking treatment and the explanation is tenuous, or there is absence of any evidence of splashing.

(i) Refer the child to the paediatric team for admission if nonaccidental injury is possible, however trivial the burn (see page 274).

FOLLOW-UP MANAGEMENT

(1) Repeat the dressing after 2 days to check the area is pain free and clean, but omit the silver sulphadiazine.

(2) Thereafter, change the dressing every 5 days, unless the wound becomes painful, smells or the bandage becomes

soaked ('strike through'), when the dressing should be renewed immediately.

(i)   When changing the dressing, leave the paraffin-impregnated gauze in place if it has become adherent to the skin, to avoid destroying the delicate new epithelium forming underneath.

(ii)   Otherwise replace the paraffin-impregnated gauze, the gauze and cotton-wool absorbent layer and the crêpe bandage.

(3) When the wound is healing and has become epithelialised it can be left exposed or covered with a dry, nonadherent dressing, e.g. Melolin.

(4) Refer burns that have not healed in 10–12 days to a plastic surgery unit for review and consideration for skin grafting.

(5) Warn the patient that healed burns will be hypersensitive, will have dry, scaly skin and may be depigmented in dark-skinned races.

MINOR BURNS OF THE HAND

(1) These are difficult to dress. Cover the hand with silver sulphadiazine cream and place the hand inside a sterile polythene bag, bandaged over a gauze ring as a seal at the wrist.

(2) The hand is then elevated and the patient is encouraged to move the fingers and use the hand.

(3) Give tetanus prophylaxis and analgesics.

(4) Replace the silver sulphadiazine cream and bag daily, as turbid fluid collects in the bag.

MINOR BURNS OF THE FACE

(1) These should be left alone and exposed to dry. They will heal in 10 days.

(2) Exclude corneal damage by staining with fluorescein.

(3) Warn the patient that alarming facial swelling may develop the following day.

ELECTROCUTION AND ELECTRICAL BURNS

These may be considered in three groups:
 (1) electrical flash burns;
 (2) low-voltage electrocution;
 (3) high-voltage injuries.

ELECTRICAL FLASH BURNS

DIAGNOSIS

 (1) These burns are caused by electrical arcing that generates brief high temperatures that may ignite clothing.
 (2) They are usually superficial partial-thickness, but may be deep dermal or even full-thickness.

MANAGEMENT

 (1) Assess the depth and extent of the burn.
 (2) Check the eyes for evidence of corneal injury, using fluorescein.
 (3) Dress the areas as for a thermal burn and treat accordingly (see page 173).

LOW-VOLTAGE ELECTROCUTION

DIAGNOSIS

 (1) Alternating current (AC) is more dangerous than direct current (DC), typically causing tetanic muscle spasm and cardiac arrhythmias.
 (2) Injury usually occurs through carelessness or faulty electrical equipment, or to inquisitive children.
 (3) The charge causes an entry wound that is often full-thickness, with potential underlying thermal tissue damage that may be extensive and include blood vessels and muscle. There is a similar exit (earthing) burn.
 (4) If the charge crosses the heart or brain, arrhythmias including ventricular fibrillation and unconsciousness may occur.

MANAGEMENT

(1) Manage cardiac or respiratory arrest as for cardiopulmonary resuscitation (see page 2).

(2) Otherwise, give oxygen and attach a cardiac monitor and pulse oximeter to the patient. Aim for an oxygen saturation over 94%. Perform a 12-lead ECG.

(3) If there is no history of altered consciousness or cardiac arrhythmia and the neurological state and ECG are normal, the patient may then be discharged, providing there is no significant thermal soft-tissue burn.

(4) All other patients require admission, with cardiac monitoring if the ECG is abnormal or there is a history of arrhythmias.

    (i)   Give intravenous normal saline for hypotension, aiming for a urine output of 100 ml/h if there is evidence of myoglobinuria (tea-coloured urine with a false positive urine dipstick test for blood).

    (ii)   Request a CT head scan if there is coma, confusion or focal neurological signs.

Note: remember that electrical burns look deceptively innocent. A white blister or small area of broken skin may cover extensive deep-tissue damage on examination.

HIGH-VOLTAGE INJURIES

DIAGNOSIS

(1) These injuries occur from electric shocks greater than 1000 volts such as from lightning, pylons, electric train cables, etc. They are very serious injuries, often fatal.

(2) The victim's clothes may ignite or explode as the current arcs over the skin.

(3) Tetanic muscle spasm occurs, causing:

    (i)   direct long-bone fracture, vertebral crush fracture and muscle tears;

    (ii)   indirect injury from falling;

    (iii) asphyxia from respiratory paralysis.

(4) The charge itself causes entry and exit wounds, which may be multiple if the charge jumps along the skin. The resultant tissue damage is deep and extensive, often requiring limb amputation.

(5) According to the pathway the charge follows, other effects include:

(i) *Heart*: cardiac arrest or arrhythmia.

(ii) *Brain*: confusion, coma, cerebral haemorrhage, spinal cord damage and peripheral nerve damage.

(iii) *Eyes and ears*: dilated pupils, uveitis, vitreous haemorrhage, ruptured ear drum, deafness and the late development of cataracts.

(iv) *Visceral and connective tissue*: immediate damage to nerves, muscles and bone from heat and vascular thrombosis or later secondary haemorrhage.

MANAGEMENT

(1) Assess the airway, give oxygen and commence cardiopulmonary resuscitation if there is no pulse or absent respirations.

(2) Otherwise, attach an ECG monitor and pulse oximeter to the patient, examine for major injuries and send blood for FBC, U&E, blood sugar, CK, G&S and blood gases.

(3) Commence an intravenous infusion, guided by the blood pressure and urine output. Fluid requirements are higher than they would appear from an assessment of the burnt areas alone.

(i) Aim for a urine output of 100 ml/h if there is myoglobinuria from rhabdomyolysis.

(4) Request a cervical spine x-ray, CXR and pelvic or limb x-rays, according to the suspected injuries.

(5) Refer patients to the surgical team for admission or referral to a specialist burns unit. Escharotomy, fasciotomy, surgical debridement and limb amputation may all be necessary.

CHEMICAL BURNS

DIAGNOSIS

(1) These occur at home, in schools, laboratories or in industrial accidents.

(2) Most agents are strong acids or alkalis, although occasionally phosphorus and phenol are responsible.

(3) Alkali burns are generally more serious than acid as they penetrate deeper.

MANAGEMENT

(1) In the first instance treat by copious irrigation with running water and wear gloves to remove any contaminated clothing. Continue irrigating for at least 20 min.

(2) Do not attempt to neutralise the chemical as most resultant reactions produce heat and will exacerbate the injury, except in the case of hydrofluoric acid.

(3) *Hydrofluoric acid burns*:
   These should be neutralised as follows:
   (i)   Conversion of hydrofluoric acid to the calcium salt is not associated with heat production and is achieved by covering the area with dressings soaked in 10% calcium gluconate solution, or by rubbing in commercially available 2.5% calcium gluconate gel (Hydrofluoric Acid Burn Jelly).
   (ii)   If the pain and burning persist, subcutaneous 10% calcium gluconate injection is advocated.
   (iii) Hypocalcaemia, hypomagnesaemia and hyperkalaemia leading to cardiac arrest may follow absorption of the fluoride ion by the skin, from as little as a 2% body surface area burn with concentrated 70% hydrofluoric acid.

(4) Refer all patients to the surgical team unless the area burnt is minimal and pain free.

(5) Remember advice is always available from the Poisons Information Centres (see page 67).

BITUMEN BURNS

DIAGNOSIS AND MANAGEMENT

(1) Road-laying and roofing accidents are usually responsible.
(2) Irrigate the area immediately with cold water.
(3) Leave the black bitumen alone and cover it with paraffin-impregnated gauze.
(4) Await blister formation or re-epithelialisation, which will allow the bitumen to drop off.
(5) Assess subsequently for the depth of the burn, which is usually partial-thickness.

THE ACUTE ABDOMEN

The aim is to resuscitate critically ill patients and to distinguish between patients requiring surgical or medical referral and patients who could be allowed home.

IMMEDIATE MANAGEMENT OF SERIOUSLY ILL PATIENTS

(1) Clear the airway, give oxygen and attach a cardiac monitor and pulse oximeter to the patient.
(2) Check the temperature, pulse, blood pressure and respiratory rate.
(3) Obtain a brief history of the onset, duration, nature and character of the pain, prior episodes of pain, relevant previous operations and illnesses, present medication and known drug allergies.
(4) Examine the chest and heart, then lay the patient flat to examine the abdomen including the femoral pulses.
(5) Consider ruptured aortic aneurysm, pancreatitis, mesenteric infarction or inferior myocardial infarction in shocked patients with acute abdominal pain.
(6) Perform a rectal examination and catheterise the bladder. Test the urine for sugar, blood, protein, bile and urobilinogen and send for microscopy and culture.

(7) Commence an intravenous infusion with normal saline. Arrange insertion of a CVP line by an experienced doctor in older patients with pre-existing cardiac disease, to avoid precipitating heart failure from fluid overload.

(8) Send blood for FBC, U&E, blood sugar, amylase and cross-match if haemorrhage is suspected. Send blood cultures if pyrexial. Check arterial blood gases.

(9) Record an ECG and request an erect CXR or lateral decubitus abdominal film if the patient is unable to sit upright, to look for free gas.

(10) Insert a nasogastric tube if there is evidence of intestinal obstruction, ileus or peritonitis.

(11) Commence broad-spectrum antibiotics such as ampicillin 1 g i.v., gentamicin 80 mg i.v. and metronidazole 500 mg i.v. for generalised peritonitis.

(12) Refer the patient immediately to the surgical team.

MANAGEMENT OF STABLE PATIENTS WITH AN ACUTE ABDOMEN

(1) *History*:
- (i)   Onset and nature of the pain:
  - (a) Explosive and excruciating pain: consider myocardial infarction, ruptured aortic aneurysm, perforated viscus, biliary or renal colic.
  - (b) Rapid, severe and constant pain: consider pancreatitis, strangulated bowel, mesenteric infarction and ectopic pregnancy.
  - (c) Gradual, steady pain: consider cholecystitis, appendicitis, diverticulitis, hepatitis and salpingitis.
  - (d) Intermittent pain with crescendos: consider mechanical obstruction.
- (ii) Location and radiation of pain:
  - (a) Central abdominal pain radiating to the back suggests an aortic aneurysm or pancreatitis.
  - (b) Flank pain radiating to the genitalia suggests ureteric colic, or rarely ruptured aortic aneurysm.

      (c) Otherwise pain tends to localise over the organ affected, provided there is peritoneal involvement, with radiation to a shoulder tip if the diaphragm is irritated, e.g. by cholecystitis or a ruptured spleen.

(iii) Associated nausea and vomiting:
      (a) Pain tends to precede the nausea and vomiting in the surgical acute abdomen.
      (b) If the nausea and vomiting precede the pain, a medical condition such as gastroenteritis or gastritis is more likely.

(iv) Fever and rigors:
      (a) A low-grade pyrexia is usual in appendicitis or diverticulitis.
      (b) A high fever and rigors suggest cholecystitis or cholangitis, diffuse peritonitis, pyelonephritis or acute salpingitis.

(2) *Examination*:
(i) Check the temperature, pulse, blood pressure and respiratory rate.
(ii) Inspect for visible peristalsis and distension, palpate for local tenderness, guarding and masses, percuss for free gas and listen for increased or absent bowel sounds.
(iii) Always perform a rectal examination, external genitalia examination in the male, and consider a vaginal examination in the female patient.
(iv) Make a careful examination of the hernial orifices, particularly in cases of intestinal obstruction.

(3) *Investigations*:
(i) Send a baseline FBC, U&E, blood sugar and amylase, although their actual value in differentiating between the various conditions is limited.
(ii) Test the urine for sugar, blood, protein, bile and urobilinogen, and send for microscopy and culture in suspected UTI.
(iii) Perform a pregnancy test in females with undiagnosed abdominal pain.
(iv) Radiology. Request:

(a) An erect CXR. This may show evidence of pulmonary disease, a secondary pleural reaction from intra-abdominal disease and free gas under the diaphragm indicating a perforation.

(b) Erect and supine abdomen films. These often confirm a diagnosis but rarely show completely unsuspected findings. Look specifically at the gas pattern, splenic shadow, renal outlines and psoas shadows, and for calcification and opacities.

(4) *Pain relief*:

    (i) Give all patients intravenous analgesia as required, such as morphine 2.5–5 mg i.v. with metoclopramide 10 mg i.v.

    (i) This does not interfere with the surgical diagnosis, which may even be facilitated.[7]

(5) *Surgical referral*. Refer all cases to the surgical team if an acute surgical condition is suspected or cannot be excluded.

CAUSES OF ACUTE ABDOMINAL PAIN

These are considered under the following headings:

(1) Intestinal disorders:
    (i) acute appendicitis;
    (ii) intestinal obstruction;
    (iii) intussusception;
    (iv) perforation of a viscus;
    (v) diverticulitis;
    (vi) gastroenteritis;
    (vii) inflammatory bowel disease.

(2) Biliary and hepatic disorders:
    (i) biliary colic;
    (ii) acute cholecystitis;
    (iii) hepatitis.

(3) Vascular disorders:
    (i) ruptured aortic aneurysm;
    (ii) ischaemic colitis;
    (iii) mesenteric infarction;

       (iv)   ruptured spleen.
(4) Pancreatic disorder:
       (i)   acute pancreatitis.
(5) Urinary disorders:
       (i)   renal and ureteric colic;
       (ii)   pyelonephritis;
       (iii) acute urinary retention;
       (iv) acute epididymo-orchitis;
       (v)   acute testicular torsion.
(6) Peritoneal and retroperitoneal disorders:
       (i)   primary peritonitis;
       (ii)   retroperitoneal haemorrhage.
(7) Gynaecological disorders:
       (i)   ruptured ectopic pregnancy;
       (ii)   acute salpingitis;
       (iii) ruptured ovarian cyst;
       (iv) torsion of an ovarian tumour;
       (v)   endometriosis.
(8) Medical disorders presenting as acute abdominal pain:
       (i)   thoracic;
       (ii)   abdominal;
       (iii) endocrine and metabolic;
       (iv) neurogenic;
       (v)   skeletal;
       (vi) psychiatric.

ACUTE APPENDICITIS

DIAGNOSIS

(1) Acute appendicitis causes poorly localised central abdominal pain, worse on coughing or moving, that classically shifts to the right iliac fossa. There is associated anorexia, nausea, vomiting and diarrhoea or constipation.
(2) A low-grade pyrexia, localised abdominal tenderness and guarding are found.
(3) A rectal examination will help diagnose a retrocaecal or pelvic appendix.
(4) The diagnosis is most difficult in the young, the elderly or the pregnant patient.

MANAGEMENT

(1) Admit all patients under the surgical team if the diagnosis is definite. Give a metronidazole suppository 1 g p.r. if rupture is suspected.

(2) Refer other suspected or atypical cases to the surgical team, e.g. the confused elderly patient, the infant with diarrhoea or the older child off his food, all of whom could have appendicitis.

INTESTINAL OBSTRUCTION

DIAGNOSIS

(1) Intermittent colicky abdominal pain occurs with abdominal distension and vomiting in high obstruction, and constipation with failure to pass flatus in low obstruction.

(2) The causes are many, including an obstructed hernia, adhesions, volvulus, intussusception, carcinoma, mesenteric infarction and Crohn's disease.

(3) Visible peristalsis may be seen, associated with tinkling bowel sounds and signs of dehydration.

(4) Always examine the hernial orifices and perform a rectal examination.

(5) Request erect and supine abdominal x-rays.
  - (i) Small bowel obstruction:
    - (a) X-rays show an empty colon and central dilated small bowel recognised by regular transverse bands (*valvulae conniventes*) extending across the entire diameter of the bowel.
    - (b) Fluid levels should be seen (but also occur in severe gastroenteritis). Over 5 are considered significant.
  - (ii) Large bowel obstruction: x-rays show peripheral dilated large bowel, with irregular haustral folds.

(6) If strangulation occurs (most common with a femoral hernia) the pain becomes more continuous and generalised, associated with tachycardia and signs of shock.

MANAGEMENT

(1) Check FBC, U&E, and blood sugar, and commence an intravenous infusion of normal saline to correct the dehydration from vomiting and fluid loss into the bowel.

(2) Pass a nasogastric tube.

(3) Refer the patient to the surgical team.

INTUSSUSCEPTION

DIAGNOSIS

(1) Intermittent abdominal pain with sudden screaming and pallor occurs in children aged 3–18 months followed by vomiting.

(2) Abdominal distension and a mass may be felt, with bloodstained mucus ('red currant jelly') found on rectal examination in 50%.

(3) Request erect and supine abdominal x-rays to look for signs of intestinal obstruction.

MANAGEMENT

(1) Insert an intravenous cannula and send blood for FBC, U&E and blood sugar.

(2) Commence careful intravenous rehydration.

(3) Refer the patient to the surgical team.

PERFORATION OF A VISCUS

DIAGNOSIS

(1) Perforation may occur anywhere in the gastrointestinal tract. Common sites are a peptic ulcer, the appendix or in a diverticulum.

(2) There may be an antecedent history of alcohol or non-steroidal anti-inflammatory drug ingestion, dyspepsia or lower abdominal pain, but perforation can occur *de novo*.

(3) It presents with severe pain and signs of generalised peritonitis with board-like rigidity. Shock soon supervenes.

(4) An erect CXR will show gas under the diaphragm in over 70% of cases.

MANAGEMENT

(1) Send blood for FBC, U&E, blood sugar and amylase, and treat shock with intravenous saline.
(2) Pass a nasogastric tube.
(3) Commence broad-spectrum antibiotics such as ampicillin 1 g i.v., gentamicin 80 mg i.v. and metronidazole 500 mg i.v.
(4) Refer the patient immediately to the surgical team.

DIVERTICULITIS

DIAGNOSIS

(1) This causes lower abdominal pain radiating to the left iliac fossa and bloody diarrhoea, sometimes with sudden profuse rectal bleeding.
(2) There is a low-grade fever, abdominal tenderness and guarding on the left with a palpable mass.
(3) Complications of perforation, severe bleeding, fistula formation and bowel obstruction may occur.

MANAGEMENT

(1) Send blood for FBC, U&E, blood sugar and G&S, and request an ECG and an erect CXR if perforation is suspected.
(2) Commence an intravenous infusion to treat shock.
(3) Refer the patient to the surgical team for bed rest and antibiotic therapy in uncomplicated cases, or for surgery in the remainder.

GASTROENTERITIS

See also 'Gastrointestinal tract infections' page 92.

DIAGNOSIS

(1) Nausea, vomiting and diarrhoea tend to precede the pain. Close contacts may be similarly affected.
(2) There is generalised abdominal discomfort, usually without localising signs of peritonism or guarding.
(3) In severe cases, an erect abdominal film will show fluid levels.

MANAGEMENT

(1) If the patient is unwell or dehydrated (particularly children), send blood for FBC, U&E, blood sugar and blood culture. Commence an intravenous infusion and refer to the medical team.
(2) Otherwise, discharge the patient with an oral glucose-electrolyte solution such as Dioralyte or Rehidrat. If symptoms persist, ask the patient to return and then send stool cultures to the laboratory.

INFLAMMATORY BOWEL DISEASE

DIAGNOSIS

(1) Ulcerative colitis associated with bouts of diarrhoea with blood stained mucus may present as a fulminating attack with fever, tachycardia, hypotension and a dilated colon on plain abdominal x-ray (i.e. toxic megacolon greater than 6 cm in diameter).
(2) Crohn's disease, associated with recurrent abdominal pain, diarrhoea, malaise and perianal fistulae or abscesses, may present acutely with obstruction, perforation or right iliac fossa pain. This can mimic acute appendicitis

MANAGEMENT

(1) Send blood for FBC, U&E, blood sugar, blood culture and commence an intravenous infusion for shock.
(2) Refer all cases to the surgical team with shock, fever, peritonitis, severe bleeding and a dilated or obstructed bowel on abdominal x-ray.

BILIARY COLIC

DIAGNOSIS

(1) Discrete episodes of colicky pain occur in the right hypochondrium, referred to the scapula.
(2) Examination reveals right upper quadrant tenderness and possibly signs of jaundice with yellow sclerae and bilirubin in the urine, if the common bile duct is obstructed.

MANAGEMENT

(1) Refer the patient to the surgical team if the pain is severe or acute cholecystitis is suspected.
(2) Otherwise refer the patient to surgical outpatients for investigation by upper abdominal ultrasound, etc.

ACUTE CHOLECYSTITIS

DIAGNOSIS

(1) Acute, constant right upper quadrant pain referred to the scapula occurs, with anorexia, nausea and vomiting.
(2) Localised tenderness is usual, sometimes with a palpable gall bladder and fever.

MANAGEMENT

(1) Send blood for FBC, U&E, blood sugar and blood culture, and commence an intravenous infusion of saline.
(2) Give ampicillin 1 g i.v. plus gentamicin 80 mg i.v. and pethidine 0.5–1 mg/kg i.v. slowly.
(3) Refer the patient to the surgical team for bed rest, analgesics, antibiotics and cholecystectomy.

HEPATITIS

DIAGNOSIS

(1) Hepatitis presents with anorexia, nausea, vomiting, malaise and joint pain.

(2) A raised temperature, jaundice, tender hepatomegaly and splenomegaly are found.
(3) Urinalysis reveals bilirubin and urobilinogen.
(4) Causes include:
  (i) Viruses, e.g. enterically transmitted hepatitis A or E, or parenterally spread hepatitis B, C or D, and infectious mononucleosis.
  (ii) Bacteria, as in leptospirosis.
  (iii) Toxins, such as alcohol and drugs including methyldopa, isoniazid and paracetamol (remember the possibility of acute poisoning).

MANAGEMENT

(1) Refer patients to the medical team with persistent vomiting, dehydration, encephalopathy or a bleeding tendency with a prolonged prothrombin time.
(2) Otherwise send diagnostic bloods for liver function tests and viral studies for hepatitis A, B or C.
(3) Advise the patient to avoid preparing food for others and to use his or her own knife, fork, spoon, cup and plate (assuming the patient could have hepatitis A or E).
(4) Advise the patient to avoid alcohol.
(5) Give the patient a referral letter to medical outpatients for definitive diagnosis and follow-up.

RUPTURED AORTIC ANEURYSM

DIAGNOSIS

(1) This classically presents with sudden abdominal pain radiating to the back or groin, faintness, collapse or unexplained shock.
(2) Abdominal examination ranges from a pulsatile tender mass, to a vague fullness and discomfort. Tachycardia and hypotension occur in 50% of cases.
(3) The diagnosis must always be considered in males over 55 years in particular, even when only one feature of the classic triad of abdominal or back pain, shock and a pulsatile or tender abdominal mass is present.

MANAGEMENT

(1) Give the patient oxygen by face mask, and record the ECG as ischaemic heart disease is usually associated or is exacerbated by the hypotension.

(2) Send blood for FBC, U&E, blood sugar, amylase and cross-match 10 units of blood and commence an intravenous infusion via a large-bore cannula.

   (i)   Give normal saline or a colloid such as polygeline (Haemaccel) cautiously to a systolic BP of no more than 90 mmHg.

   (ii) Aim for rapid surgical control rather than massive pre-operative transfusion.

(3) Catheterise the bladder.

(4) Refer the patient urgently to the surgical team for immediate laparotomy. Contact the anaesthetist and warn theatre.

(5) If the diagnosis is in doubt and only if the patient is stable, consider an ultrasound scan to confirm the presence of an aneurysm, or a CT scan that will also demonstrate if it has ruptured.

(6) Otherwise, proceed directly to theatre. Apply a pneumatic antishock garment such as MAST if the patient remains severely hypotensive, particularly if interhospital transfer is necessary.

ISCHAEMIC COLITIS

DIAGNOSIS

This usually occurs in an elderly patient with recurrent abdominal pain, progressing to episodes of bloody diarrhoea or intestinal obstruction from stricture formation.

MANAGEMENT

(1) Send blood for FBC, U&E, blood sugar and G&S if there is shock and commence an intravenous infusion.

(2) Record the ECG.

(3) Perform an abdominal x-ray to look for 'thumb printing' of the colonic wall and proximal dilatation.

(4) Refer the patient to the surgical team.

MESENTERIC INFARCTION

DIAGNOSIS

(1) Sudden onset of severe, diffuse abdominal pain occurs, usually in an elderly patient, associated with vomiting and bloody diarrhoea.

(2) Abdominal distension, tenderness, shock, absent bowel sounds and rectal bleeding supervene.

MANAGEMENT

(1) Send blood for FBC, U&E, blood sugar, cross-match 2–4 units of blood and commence an intravenous infusion.

(2) Record the ECG.

(3) Refer the patient to the surgical team, who will determine the need for angiography to confirm the diagnosis.

RUPTURED SPLEEN

DIAGNOSIS

(1) Left lower rib injuries following blunt trauma are associated with splenic damage in up to 20% of cases.

(2) Occasionally trivial injury to an enlarged spleen in glandular fever, malaria or leukaemia may cause rupture.

(3) Rupture may be *acute*, causing tachycardia, hypotension and abdominal tenderness with referred pain to the left shoulder.

(4) Or rupture may be *delayed*, occurring up to 2 weeks or more after an episode of trauma. Initial localised discomfort and referred shoulder tip pain give way to signs of intra-abdominal haemorrhage.

MANAGEMENT

(1) Send a FBC and cross-match 6 units of blood for an acutely ruptured spleen. Commence a rapid intravenous infusion and refer the patient immediately to the surgical team.

(2) In the absence of shock, insert an intravenous cannula for a delayed rupture of a subcapsular haematoma and send blood for a FBC and G&S.
  (i)   Arrange an urgent upper abdominal ultrasound or CT scan.
  (ii) Delayed splenic rupture is also supported by a CXR showing fractured left lower ribs and a basal pleural effusion, and an abdominal x-ray showing a displaced stomach bubble to the right and an enlarged soft-tissue shadow in the splenic area.
(3) Refer the patient to the surgical team for admission.

ACUTE PANCREATITIS

DIAGNOSIS

(1) Predisposing factors include alcohol abuse and gall stones.
(2) Acute pancreatitis presents with sudden, severe abdominal pain radiating to the back, eased by sitting forward, associated with repeated vomiting or retching (unlike a perforated peptic ulcer).
(3) Tachycardia with hypotension, a low-grade fever and epigastric tenderness, guarding and decreased or absent bowel sounds are found.

MANAGEMENT

(1) Send blood for FBC, U&E, blood sugar, calcium, amylase and G&S. Commence an intravenous infusion of normal saline and pass a nasogastric tube.
(2) Check the blood gases.
(3) Record the ECG that may show diffuse T wave inversion, in the absence of myocardial ischaemia.
(4) Refer the patient to the surgical team. A raised serum lipase is more sensitive and specific than an amylase, and may become the preferred test although neither is pathognomic of pancreatitis.

RENAL AND URETERIC COLIC

DIAGNOSIS

(1) Sudden, severe colicky pain radiating from the loin to the genitalia, associated with restlessness, vomiting and sweating is characteristic.
(2) There may be urinary frequency and haematuria.
(3) Loin tenderness in the costovertebral angle may be found and urinalysis shows macroscopic or microscopic haematuria.
(4) Always consider a possible ruptured abdominal aortic aneurysm in males over 55 years with a first episode of renal colic, especially if haematuria is absent (see page 189).

MANAGEMENT

(1) Check FBC, U&E and send the urine for microscopy and culture.
(2) Treat pain:
    (i)   Use diclofenac (Voltarol) 75 mg i.m. It is as effective as pethidine, is not a controlled drug and should discourage those who are only seeking narcotics.
    (ii)   Alternatively, pethidine 0.5–1 mg/kg slowly i.v. is the traditional analgesic, given with an antiemetic.
(3) A plain abdominal x-ray KUB view (kidneys, ureters, bladder) may show a calculus in the line of the renal tract. An IVU is essential to confirm the diagnosis.
(4) Refer the patient to the surgical team.

PYELONEPHRITIS

DIAGNOSIS

(1) This presents with frequency, dysuria, malaise, nausea, vomiting and sometimes rigors.
(2) Raised temperature, renal angle tenderness and vague low abdominal pain are found.

(3) Dipstick urinalysis shows blood and protein. Urine microscopy shows bacteria, leucocytes and red blood cells.

MANAGEMENT

(1) Send FBC, U&E, blood sugar, blood culture and a urine culture for any patient who is significantly ill:
  (i) This should include patients with vomiting, dehydration, or prostration; those who are pregnant, very young or old; and those who are known to have urinary tract abnormalities, e.g. a duplex system, horseshoe kidney or renal/ureteric stones.
  (ii) Commence gentamicin 80 mg i.v. and refer these patients to the surgical team for admission.
(2) Otherwise, if the symptoms are mild and consistent with predominant cystitis, send a urine culture and commence an oral antibiotic such as trimethoprim 200 mg b.d. for 1 week.
(3) Return the patient to their general practitioner, with a letter requesting the GP to repeat the urine culture after the antibiotics, to ensure that the infection has been eradicated.
(4) Any male with a proven UTI must subsequently be referred to urology outpatients for investigation.

ACUTE URINARY RETENTION

DIAGNOSIS

(1) Predisposing factors include prostatic hypertrophy, urethral stricture, pelvic neoplasm, constipation in the elderly, anticholinergic drugs and pregnancy. Occasionally retention is due to a neurogenic cause such as multiple sclerosis.
(2) The enlarged bladder is easily palpable, dull to percussion and is usually painful, although in the semiconscious patient it may manifest as restlessness.
(3) Always perform a rectal examination and assess perineal sensation in all patients.

MANAGEMENT

(1) This depends on the suspected aetiology.

(2) Send blood for FBC, U&E and blood sugar.

(3) If the patient is in pain, carefully pass a urethral catheter by a strict aseptic procedure, and send a specimen of urine for culture.

(4) Refer the patient to the surgical team or gynaecologists as appropriate.

ACUTE EPIDIDYMO-ORCHITIS

DIAGNOSIS

(1) This occurs in sexually active men with a preceding history of urethritis, or after urinary tract instrumentation including catheterisation.

(2) Pain begins gradually, usually localised to the epididymis or testis associated with a low-grade fever.

(3) Urine microscopy shows leucocytes and there may be a raised white cell count in the blood.

MANAGEMENT

(1) *Never* diagnose epididymo-orchitis in a patient under 25 years old without considering testicular torsion first.

(2) If torsion has been excluded, send urine for culture and give the patient a scrotal support, analgesics such as paracetamol 500 mg and codeine phosphate 8 mg (co-codamol) 2 tablets q.d.s. and an antibiotic.

(3) The choice of antibiotic depends on the suspected aetiology:

    (i) Bacterial cystitis with epididymitis requires trimethoprim 200 mg orally b.d. for 1 week and referral to a urology clinic.

    (ii) Nonspecific urethritis with epididymitis requires doxycycline 100 mg orally b.d. for 10 days and follow-up in a genitourinary medicine clinic.

    (iii) Suspected gonococcal urethritis with epididymitis should ideally be treated from the outset by a genitourinary medicine clinic.

ACUTE TESTICULAR TORSION

DIAGNOSIS

(1) Suspect this diagnosis in any male under 25 years old with sudden pain in a testicle that may radiate to the lower abdomen. There may be associated nausea and vomiting.
(2) The testicle lies horizontally and high in the scrotum, and is very tender. There may be a small hydrocoele.
(3) Urinalysis is typically negative and a white cell count normal.

MANAGEMENT

(1) Always refer all cases urgently to the surgical team as the testicle becomes nonviable after 6 h of torsion.
(2) Even if more than 6 h have elapsed, still refer the patient for surgery as orchidopexy is required on the other side, to prevent subsequent torsion there.

PRIMARY PERITONITIS

DIAGNOSIS

(1) Primary bacterial peritonitis occurs almost exclusively in patients with ascites, particularly due to cirrhosis or the nephrotic syndrome.
(2) Fever, abdominal pain and tenderness occur.

MANAGEMENT

(1) Send FBC, U&E, LFTs, blood sugar and blood cultures.
(2) Refer the patient to the medical team for diagnostic peritoneal tap and culture, to exclude *Mycobacterium tuberculosis* and to distinguish bacterial peritonitis from familial Mediterranean fever.

RETROPERITONEAL HAEMORRHAGE

DIAGNOSIS

(1) This condition may occur following trauma to the pelvis, kidney or back, from aortic aneurysm rupture, or from trivial trauma — even spontaneously in those with a bleeding tendency or on anticoagulants.
(2) It presents with hypovolaemic shock following trauma, in the absence of an obvious external or internal thoracic or abdominal source for haemorrhage. A paralytic ileus may develop.
(3) Plain abdominal x-ray will show loss of the psoas shadow and possibly fractures of the vertebral transverse processes in traumatic cases.

MANAGEMENT

(1) Send blood for FBC, U&E, blood sugar, amylase and cross-match blood according to the degree of shock.
(2) Insert a wide-bore intravenous cannula and begin crystalloid infusion with normal saline.
(3) Check the urine for blood. If present, request an urgent IVU to exclude renal damage.
(4) Refer the patient to the surgical team. An abdominal CT scan will localise the bleeding in most cases.

RUPTURED ECTOPIC PREGNANCY

See page 343.

ACUTE SALPINGITIS

See page 344.

RUPTURED OVARIAN CYST

See page 345.

TORSION OF AN OVARIAN TUMOUR

See page 346.

ENDOMETRIOSIS

See page 346.

MEDICAL DISORDERS PRESENTING AS ACUTE ABDOMINAL PAIN

It is rare for nonsurgical causes of acute abdominal pain to present without other symptoms or signs suggesting their true origin. Always remember diabetic ketoacidosis, diagnosed by finding glycosuria and ketonuria on urinalysis (see page 35). Causes include:

(1) *Thoracic origin*:
- (i)   Myocardial infarction, pericarditis.
- (ii)   Pulmonary embolus, pleurisy.
- (iii)   Aortic dissection.

(2) *Abdominal origin*:
- (i)   Pancreatitis.
- (ii)   Hepatic congestion from hepatitis or right heart failure.
- (iii)   Intestinal ischaemia from atheroma or sickle cell disease, vasculitis and Henoch–Schönlein purpura.
- (iv)   Constipation, particularly in the elderly.
- (v)   Infection including gastroenteritis, pyelonephritis and primary peritonitis.

(3) *Endocrine and metabolic origin*:
- (i)   Diabetic ketoacidosis.
- (ii)   Addison's disease.
- (iii)   Hypercalcaemia — 'stones, bones and abdominal groans'.
- (iv)   Porphyria (acute intermittent).
- (v)   Lead poisoning, paracetamol or iron poisoning.

(4) *Neurogenic origin*:
- (i)   Herpes zoster.
- (ii)   Tabes dorsalis.
- (iii)   Radiculitis from spinal cord degeneration or malignancy.

(5) *Skeletal origin*: collapsed vertebra due to osteoporosis, neoplasm or infection e.g. tuberculosis.

(6) *Psychiatric*: Munchausen's syndrome or 'hospital hopper'.

(i) Be suspicious of patients with multiple abdominal scars acquired at other hospitals, probably not living locally and with no general practitioner, who present with acute abdominal pain or renal colic.

(ii) Their aim is to gain hospital admission or narcotic analgesics by feigning illness.

(iii) Ask for a previous hospital number or admission details, so you can 'go and verify their story'. If this does not prompt them to leave of their own accord, seek advice from a senior doctor.

MANAGEMENT

This list is long and exhaustive. A careful history and examination, and request for FBC, U&E, LFTs, blood sugar, amylase, urinalysis, ECG, CXR and abdominal x-ray will avoid missing the more serious diagnoses.

REFERENCES

1   Teasdale G.M., Murray G., Anderson E. *et al.* (1990). Risks of acute traumatic intracranial haematoma in children and adults: implications for managing head injuries. *British Medical Journal*; **300**:363–367.

2   Gentleman D., Dearden M., Midgley S., Maclean D. (1993). Guidelines for resuscitation and transfer of patients with serious head injury. *British Medical Journal*; **307**:547–552.

3   Woodring J., Lee C., Jenkins K. (1988). Spinal fractures in blunt chest trauma. *Journal of Trauma*; **28**:789–793.

4   Champion H., Danne P., Finelli F. (1986). Emergency thoracotomy. *Archives of Emergency Medicine*; **3**:95–9

5   Frankel H., Rozycki G., Ochsner G. *et al.* (1994). Indications for obtaining surveillance thoracic and lumbar spine radiographs. *Journal of Trauma*; **37**:673–676.

6   Langford R.M., Armstrong R.F. (1989). Algorithm for managing injury from smoke inhalation. *British Medical Journal*; **299**:902–905.

7   Attard A., Corlett M., Kidner N. *et al.* (1992). Safety of early pain relief for acute abdominal pain. *British Medical Journal*; **305**:554–556.

ORTHOPAEDIC EMERGENCIES

INJURIES TO THE SHOULDER AND UPPER ARM

FRACTURES OF THE CLAVICLE

DIAGNOSIS

(1) These fractures are usually due to direct violence or to transmitted force from a fall on to the outstretched hand. In children a greenstick fracture is common; in adults, a fracture between the middle and outer thirds.

(2) There is tenderness and local deformity. An AP x-ray of the shoulder usually shows the fracture clearly.

MANAGEMENT

(1) Support the weight of the arm in a triangular sling, and give an analgesic such as paracetamol 500 mg and codeine phosphate 8 mg (co-codamol) 2 tablets q.d.s.

(2) Refer the patient to the next fracture clinic.

(3) Rarely, comminuted fractures or fractures causing compression of underlying nerves or vessels may be treated operatively and should be referred immediately to the orthopaedic team.

(4) The traditional figure-of-eight bandage has generally been abandoned as it is uncomfortable and difficult to keep tight.

ACROMIOCLAVICULAR DISLOCATION

DIAGNOSIS

(1) A fall on to the shoulder that tears the acromioclavicular ligament results in subluxation, but if the strong conoid and trapezoid coracoclavicular ligaments are torn as well, dislocation occurs with the clavicle losing all connection with the scapula.

(2) Subluxation causes local tenderness, whereas full dislocation causes a prominent outer end of the clavicle and drooping of the shoulder, with pain on movement.

(3) X-ray of the acromioclavicular joint with the patient standing will show the displacement of the clavicle, which is highlighted by comparing the shoulders when the patient is holding weights in both hands.

MANAGEMENT

(1) Support subluxations in a sling. Give the patient analgesics and refer to the next fracture clinic.
(2) Discuss complete dislocations immediately with the orthopaedic team as various operations are available (none of which is entirely satisfactory).

STERNOCLAVICULAR DISLOCATION

DIAGNOSIS

(1) This dislocation is rare, caused by a considerable blow to the front of the shoulder or a fall, resulting in the inner end of the clavicle displacing forwards or backwards.
(2) Anterior displacement results in local tenderness and asymmetry of the medial ends of the clavicles.
(3) Posterior displacement may impinge on the trachea or great vessels.
(4) X-rays are not easy to interpret, although AP and oblique views should be requested. A CT scan may be required in difficult cases.

MANAGEMENT

(1) A triangular sling and analgesics are suitable for subluxations. Refer the patient to the next fracture clinic.
(2) Refer posterior dislocations causing pressure symptoms immediately to the orthopaedic team.
(3) Discuss full anterior dislocations with the orthopaedic team; as with acromioclavicular dislocations, once reduced they are difficult to hold in place.

FRACTURES OF THE SCAPULA

DIAGNOSIS

(1) These can be divided into fractures of the neck, body, spine, acromion and coracoid, and are usually due to direct trauma.

(2) Their importance is indicating that considerable trauma has been applied to the area, so a careful check for associated rib, pulmonary, spinal column and shoulder injuries must be made.

MANAGEMENT

(1) Treat the associated injuries as a priority.

(2) Otherwise use a sling, give the patient analgesics and refer to the next fracture clinic.

ANTERIOR DISLOCATION OF THE SHOULDER

DIAGNOSIS

(1) This dislocation is caused by forced abduction and external rotation of the shoulder relative to the trunk, commonest in young adults from sports or traffic accidents, or in the elderly from a fall.

(2) It tends to become recurrent, when dislocation may occur with a trivial injury, movement or even spontaneously in bed!

(3) The arm appears slightly abducted and the shoulder looks 'squared off' with a prominent acromion.

(4) The following complications occur, and must be looked for and recorded *before* any attempts at manipulation:

　(i)　Axillary (circumflex) nerve damage. This is tested by assessing for sensory loss over the upper lateral aspect of the upper arm (testing for shoulder movement by the deltoid is too painful to be meaningful).

　(ii)　Posterior cord of the brachial plexus — damage to this is assessed by testing wrist extension by the radial nerve. Rarely other parts of the brachial plexus are damaged.

(iii) Axillary artery damage. This is checked for by palpating the brachial pulse.

(iv) Fracture of the upper humerus. This must always be specifically looked for on the x-ray.

MANAGEMENT

(1) Give the patient morphine 2.5–5 mg i.v. with an antiemetic such as metoclopramide 10 mg i.v. if there is severe pain (unusual in recurrent dislocations). Reduce the dose of morphine in the elderly patient.

(2) Always x-ray the shoulder even if you are sure of the diagnosis, to avoid missing an associated humeral head fracture. Look for the following features.

(i) The humeral head is displaced medially and anteriorly with loss of contact with the glenoid fossa on the anteroposterior view.

(ii) In doubtful cases always look at the lateral view (especially if posterior dislocation has occurred — see page 206).

(iii) Look carefully for a humeral head fracture:

(a) A fracture of the greater tuberosity will not influence the initial reduction.

(b) A fracture through the humeral head or upper humerus should be referred directly to the orthopaedic team, without any attempt at reduction.

(3) Perform the reduction under general anaesthesia for fit, muscular, young patients or following a failed reduction using intravenous agents. In the elderly and for recurrent dislocations use intravenous midazolam 2.5–5 mg, provided that monitoring and resuscitation equipment are available and dentures, rings, etc. have been removed. There are two methods of reduction:

(i) *Kocher's manoeuvre.*

(a) Gentle traction is applied to the arm flexed at the elbow and then external rotation is slowly exerted.

      (b) The shoulder may 'clunk' back during exter-
nal rotation; if it does not, when 90° is
reached adduct the arm across the chest and
internally rotate it.

      (c) The shoulder is felt to slip back; if not, repeat
the whole procedure again.

  (ii) *Hippocratic method.* Traction is applied to the
straight arm gently adducted over countertraction from the physician's stockinged foot
placed in the axilla.

(4) After reduction, place the arm in a sling strapped to the
body, or enclosed under the patient's clothes, to prevent
external rotation and a recurrent dislocation. Repeat the
shoulder x-ray to confirm the reduction.

(5) Test again for neurovascular damage.

(6) Give the patient an analgesic, with instructions to keep
the arm adducted and internally rotated, and refer to the
next fracture clinic.

POSTERIOR DISLOCATION OF THE SHOULDER

DIAGNOSIS

(1) This condition is uncommon, occurring classically
during electrocution or seizures or from a direct blow
(e.g. in boxing) and is easily missed.

(2) The arm is held adducted and internally rotated and the
greater tuberosity of the humerus feels prominent.
External rotation is severely limited and painful.

MANAGEMENT

(1) Give the patient morphine 2.5–5 mg i.v. with an
antiemetic such as metoclopramide 10 mg i.v.

(2) X-rays of the shoulder must include two views as the AP
view may appear normal.

  (i) On the AP view look for the 'light bulb' sign due
to the internally rotated humerus displaying a
globular head, and for 'loss of parallelism'
between the humeral head and the glenoid fossa.

(ii)   On the axillary lateral view look for the humeral head lying behind the glenoid.

(iii)   An alternative to the axillary lateral view is the lateral scapular or 'Y' view, which is less painful as it does not require abduction of the shoulder. Again look for the humeral head displaced posterior to the glenoid.

(3) Perform the reduction using midazolam 2.5–5 mg i.v. provided that monitoring and resuscitation equipment are available.

(i)   Apply traction to the arm abducted to 90°.

(ii)   Gently externally rotate the arm.

(4) After reduction, place the arm in a sling and repeat the shoulder x-ray to confirm reduction. Occasionally the reduction may be unstable and immediate orthopaedic referral required.

(5) Give the patient an analgesic and refer to the next fracture clinic.

ROTATOR CUFF TEAR: SUPRASPINATUS RUPTURE

DIAGNOSIS

(1) Sudden traction on the arm may tear the rotator cuff, particularly supraspinatus. Other muscles forming the rotator cuff may also tear but are difficult to diagnose in the acute state.

(2) There is localised tenderness under the acromion with supraspinatus rupture and inability to initiate shoulder abduction.

MANAGEMENT

(1) Refer the young patient immediately to the orthopaedic team for consideration of operative repair.

(2) Give the elderly patient a sling and analgesics, and refer to the physiotherapy department or to the orthopaedic clinic.

FRACTURES OF THE UPPER HUMERUS

DIAGNOSIS

(1) These fractures usually occur in elderly patients and may involve the greater tuberosity, lesser tuberosity, anatomical neck or the surgical neck of the humerus.

(2) There is localised pain and loss of movement, often with dramatic bruising gravitating down the arm.

(3) Complications include:
   (i)   shoulder dislocation;
   (ii) complete distraction of the humeral head off the shaft;
   (iii) axillary (circumflex) nerve damage causing anaesthesia over the upper, lateral aspect of the upper arm and loss of deltoid movement;
   (iv) axillary vessel damage.

MANAGEMENT

(1) Refer patients immediately to the orthopaedic team with:
   (i)   a grossly angulated or totally distracted humeral head;
   (ii) fractures associated with a dislocation;
   (iii) markedly displaced greater tuberosity fractures;
   (iv) vascular damage.

(2) Otherwise, use a collar and cuff to allow gravity to exert gentle traction. Give the patient an analgesic such as paracetamol 500 mg and codeine phosphate 8 mg (co-codamol) 2 tablets q.d.s.

(3) Remember that the elderly patient may now need social services support in the form of 'meals on wheels', a home help and possibly a district nurse. Inform the general practitioner by telephone and letter so he or she may visit the patient too.

(4) Refer the patient to the fracture clinic for follow-up.

FRACTURES OF THE SHAFT OF THE HUMERUS

DIAGNOSIS

(1) These fractures are caused by direct trauma or a fall on to the outstretched hand.

(2) Upper third fractures tend to result in the proximal fragment being adducted by the pectoralis major, whereas in middle third fractures the proximal fragment is abducted by the deltoid.

(3) When x-rays are requested always include views of the shoulder and elbow. Remember the old adage to 'x-ray the joint above and the joint below any fracture'.

(4) Complications are usually seen in the middle third fractures, including:
   (i)   compound injury;
   (ii) radial nerve damage in the spiral groove, causing weak wrist extension and sensory loss over the dorsum of the thumb.

MANAGEMENT

(1) Refer immediately to the orthopaedic team patients who have grossly angulated or compound fractures, and fractures involving a radial nerve palsy, where the nerve may have been completely severed (e.g. by a severely comminuted, angulated or compound injury).

(2) Otherwise support the arm for comfort in a U-slab plaster. This should not require analgesia to apply:
   (i)   Use a 15-cm width plaster slab applied medially under the axilla, around the elbow and up over the lateral aspect of the upper arm on to the shoulder, having padded the arm well with cotton-wool.
   (ii) Hold the slab in place with a cotton bandage and support the arm in a sling.

(3) Give the patient analgesics and review in the next fracture clinic. Social services support is needed for the elderly, who may require admission if they are unable to cope.

INJURIES TO THE ELBOW AND FOREARM

SUPRACONDYLAR FRACTURE OF THE HUMERUS

DIAGNOSIS

(1) This fracture occurs most commonly in children, from a fall on to the outstretched hand, although it is seen in adults.

(2) There is tenderness and swelling over the distal humerus, but the olecranon and two epicondyles remain in their usual 'equilateral triangle' relationship (this is lost in dislocation of the elbow).

(3) There is a risk of the distal fragment displacing posteriorly, causing damage to the brachial artery on the lower end of the proximal fragment. Local tissue swelling will quickly worsen any ischaemia.

(4) Median nerve damage may also occur causing sensory loss over the radial three-and-a-half fingers and weakness of abductor pollicis.

(5) X-ray will show the displacement, although one-third of fractures are undisplaced, some merely greenstick. Comparison with views of the other normal elbow is useful if there is difficulty interpreting the radiographs.

MANAGEMENT

(1) Test for median nerve damage and look for any signs of arterial occlusion. These include pain, pallor, paralysis, paraesthesiae, pulselessness and cold. If arterial occlusion is suspected refer the patient immediately to the orthopaedic team.

(2) Even if there is no arterial damage refer all these fractures, including the comminuted type in adults to the orthopaedic team for possible admission overnight.

CONDYLAR AND EPICONDYLAR FRACTURES OF THE HUMERUS

DIAGNOSIS

(1) The lateral condyle tends to be fractured in children and the medial epicondyle at any age, due to direct violence or forced contraction of the forearm flexors that attach to it.

(2) There is pain, swelling (which may be minimal) and loss of full elbow extension if the medial epicondyle is trapped in the joint, usually following dislocation of the elbow.

(3) The ulnar nerve may be damaged, causing sensory loss over the medial one-and-a-half digits and weakness of the finger adductors and abductors.

(4) X-rays are often very difficult to interpret in children as many of the structures are still cartilaginous. Helpful clues to look for are:

    (i)   *The posterior fat-pad sign* (see Fig. 7). This indicates a joint effusion and is indirect evidence

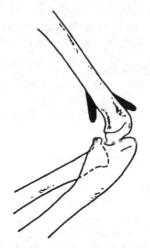

Fig. 7 Line drawing of a lateral elbow radiograph showing an anterior and posterior fat-pad sign (shaded areas) indicating a joint effusion.

of significant trauma. It is also typically seen with radial head fractures.

(ii)   Comparison with the normal elbow placed in a similar anatomical position. Look for any differences between the two sides.

(iii) The capitellum epiphysis is visible by age one year, the medial epicondyle epiphysis by age 6 years and the lateral epicondyle epiphysis appears by age 11 years. If an epiphysis which should be visible by age is missing, suspect displacement from injury.

MANAGEMENT

Refer all these fractures to the orthopaedic team. Because the structures are mainly cartilaginous, the fractures are always more extensive than they appear on the x-ray.

DISLOCATION OF THE ELBOW

DIAGNOSIS

(1) This is caused by a fall on the outstretched hand driving the olecranon posteriorly (very rarely anterior, medial or lateral displacement occurs).

(2) The normal 'equilateral triangle' between the olecranon and two epicondyles is lost (unlike the supracondylar fracture).

(3) The main complications are:
   (i)   Ulnar nerve damage causing sensory loss over the medial one-and-a-half fingers and weakness of the finger adductors, with the fingers held straight.
   (ii) Median nerve damage causing sensory loss over the radial three-and-a-half fingers and weakness of abductor pollicis.
   (iii) Brachial artery damage causing loss of the radial pulse with pain, pallor, paralysis, paraesthesiae and other signs of arterial occlusion.

(4) X-ray usually clearly shows the dislocation, but look for associated fractures of the coronoid process of the ulna or radial head in adults, and of the humeral epicondyles or lateral condyle in children.

MANAGEMENT

(1) Give the patient a sling, and intravenous analgesia for the pain.
(2) Refer all cases immediately to the orthopaedic team for reduction under a general anaesthetic.

PULLED ELBOW

DIAGNOSIS

(1) This is typical in children aged 2–6 years following traction on the arm, such as grabbing the child's arm as it runs off or falls.
(2) The radial head is subluxed out of the annular ligament causing local pain and loss of use of the arm, particularly supination. The arm is held with the elbow semi-flexed and pronated.

MANAGEMENT

(1) If there is pain localised over the radial head with limitation of supination, and the history is typical, perform the reduction without prior x-ray:
   (i) Gently flex the forearm upwards, alternately firmly supinating then pronating, with pressure applied over the radial head.
   (ii) The radial head is felt to click back; usually the child declines the offer of a sling!
(2) Otherwise x-ray the elbow in equivocal cases to avoid missing a supracondylar fracture.

FRACTURES OF THE OLECRANON

DIAGNOSIS

(1) These fractures follow a fall on to the point of the elbow or forced triceps contraction, which may then distract the olecranon leaving a palpable subcutaneous gap.
(2) There is therefore loss of active elbow extension.

(3) X-ray will show whether the fracture is displaced or merely hairline. Anterior dislocation of the elbow may accompany a displaced olecranon fracture.

MANAGEMENT

(1) Give the patient analgesics and a sling, and refer immediately to the orthopaedic team for operative reduction if there is displacement of the olecranon or an associated anterior dislocation of the elbow.
(2) Otherwise, if there is an undisplaced hairline fracture only, put the patient in a long arm plaster (with the elbow flexed) and refer to the next fracture clinic.

FRACTURES OF THE RADIAL HEAD

DIAGNOSIS

(1) These fractures are caused by direct violence or by an indirect transmitted force up the radius, which is driven against the capitellum.
(2) There is localised pain and tenderness over the radial head, and discomfort on attempted full extension and supination of the forearm.
(3) Unfortunately this injury is commonly missed, usually because it is not thought of, or because it is not seen on x-ray.
(4) It may be difficult or impossible to see a fracture on x-ray of the elbow, but look for corroborating evidence of a posterior fat-pad sign (see Fig. 7).
(5) If doubt exists, ask specifically for additional radial head views.

MANAGEMENT

(1) Refer the patient to the orthopaedic team if the radial head is comminuted or grossly displaced.
(2) Manage nondisplaced or crack fractures in a collar and cuff and refer the patient to the next fracture clinic.

(3) If there is severe localised pain, a plaster elbow backslab may be used for protection.

FRACTURES OF THE RADIAL AND ULNAR SHAFTS

These two bones tend to act as a unit, attached proximally at the radial head by the annular ligament, throughout their length by the interosseous membrane and distally by the radio-ulnar ligaments. It is rare to fracture one bone in isolation and, as in humeral shaft fractures, it is vital to x-ray the joints above and below (here, the elbow and wrist).

DIAGNOSIS

(1) Injury is caused by direct trauma or by falling on to an outstretched hand, usually with an element of rotation fracturing both bones.
(2) There is localised tenderness, deformity and sometimes compound injury.
(3) X-ray will show the fractures. If one bone is angulated but the other is apparently not fractured, look for a second dislocation injury:
    (i) *Monteggia fracture*. Fracture of the upper ulna with dislocation of the radial head.
    (ii) *Galeazzi fracture*. Fracture of the lower radius with dislocation of the inferior radio-ulnar joint at the wrist.

MANAGEMENT

(1) Refer all these difficult fractures to the orthopaedic team.
(2) In the rare instance of an isolated, undisplaced, single forearm bone fracture, place the arm in a full-arm plaster cast from the metacarpal heads to the upper arm, with the elbow flexed at a right angle and the wrist in the midposition. Refer the patient to the next fracture clinic.

INJURIES TO THE WRIST AND HAND

COLLES' FRACTURE

DIAGNOSIS

(1) This is a fracture of the distal 2.5 cm of the radius from a fall on the outstretched hand, commonest in elderly females with osteoporosis.

(2) The classical 'dinner fork' deformity is due to dorsal angulation and dorsal displacement of the distal radial fragment, which may also be impacted, radially displaced and radially tilted.

(3) X-ray demonstrates the fracture, often associated with an ulnar styloid avulsion fracture from attachment to the triangular fibrocartilage.

MANAGEMENT

(1) Undisplaced, or minimally displaced fractures particularly in the elderly may be treated directly with a Colles' backslab.

(2) Otherwise reduce the fracture under a Bier's block, axillary block, general anaesthetic or haematoma block, according to departmental policy.

(3) Intravenous regional anaesthesia or Bier's block technique:

    (i)   Two doctors are required allowing one to perform the manipulation and the other, with anaesthetic experience and prior training in the procedure, to perform the block:

        (a) at least one nurse attends to the patient, checks the blood pressure and assists the doctors;

        (b) explain the technique to the patient who should sign a written consent form.

    (ii) The technique is contraindicated in peripheral vascular disease including Raynaud's, sickle cell disease, cellulitis, uncooperative patients including children under 14, known local anaesthetic sensitivity and hypertension with systolic blood pressure over 200 mmHg.

(iii)   ECG and BP monitoring must be available in an area with full resuscitation facilities and a tipping trolley. The patient must be starved for 4 h before the procedure.

(iv)   Use a specifically designed and properly maintained single 15-cm adult cuff, checking first for leaks or malfunction. Apply the cuff to the upper arm over cotton-wool padding.

(v)   Insert a small intravenous cannula into the dorsum of the hand on the affected side and a second cannula into the other hand or wrist.

(vi)   Elevate the affected arm for 3 minutes to empty the veins, rather than using an Esmarch bandage which is generally too painful.

(vii)   Keeping the arm elevated, inflate the cuff to 300 mmHg. The radial pulse should no longer be palpable and the veins remain empty.

(viii)   Lower the arm and slowly inject 0.5% prilocaine 3 mg/kg (10 ml of 0.5% prilocaine contains 50 mg). Make a note of the time of injection.

(ix)   Continuously monitor the cuff pressure for leakage. Keep the cuff inflated for a minimum of 20 min to ensure the prilocaine is fully tissue bound, but with a maximum of 1 h.

(x)   Wait at least 5 min before performing the manipulation after confirming the adequacy of block. Request a check x-ray and repeat the manipulation immediately if reduction is unsatisfactory.

(xi)   If satisfactory, deflate the cuff then re-inflate for 2 min observing for signs of local anaesthetic toxicity, although the maximum safe dosage of prilocaine is 6 mg/kg (double the amount used in the block). Signs of local anaesthetic toxicity include:
(a)   restlessness, perioral tingling, dizziness, slurred speech;
(b)   loss of consciousness, fits, bradycardia and hypotension, which are virtually unknown with prilocaine.

(xii) The patient then rests for at least 2 h whilst regular observations are made. Allow home with an accompanying adult if the plaster is comfortable and the patient feels well.

(4) Reduction and immobilisation are achieved as follows:

(i) Prepare a 15-cm plaster slab measured from the metacarpal heads to the angle of the elbow. Cut a slot for the thumb and remove a triangle to accommodate the final ulnar deviation: see Fig. 8 (a) and (b).

(ii) Disimpact the fracture by firm traction on the thumb and fingers, whilst an assistant provides countertraction to the upper arm, keeping the elbow bent at a right angle. Also by hyperextending the wrist in the direction of deformity.

(iii) Next extend the elbow and then use your thenar eminence to reduce the dorsal displacement and to rotate back the dorsal angulation, with the heel of your other hand acting as a fulcrum.

(iv) Alter grip to push the distal fragment ulnarwards to correct radial displacement.

(v) Finally hold the hand pronated in full ulnar deviation with the wrist slightly flexed. Apply the backslab to the radial side of the forearm, which is well padded with cotton-wool: see Fig. 8 (c).

(vi) Hold the backslab in place with a cotton bandage and take a check x-ray to assess the adequacy of the reduction before terminating the anaesthetic:

(a) In a young person reduction should be perfect.

(b) In an elderly person up to 10° of residual dorsal angulation can be accepted.

(5) Give the patient a sling, with instructions to keep the shoulder and fingers moving, and review in the next fracture clinic.

(6) Remember to check that the elderly will be able to manage at home, particularly if they already rely on a walking frame. Social services help may be needed, and the general practitioner should be informed by letter and by telephone.

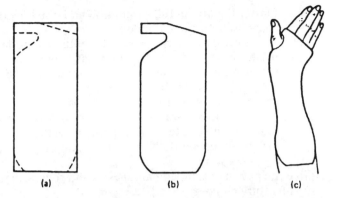

Fig. 8. The Colles' backslab plaster. (a) and (b). The backslab is prepared by trimming to permit thumb movements, full elbow flexion and to allow for the final ulnar deviation of the wrist. (c) The backslab in position.

SMITH'S FRACTURE

DIAGNOSIS

(1) This fracture is caused by a fall on to the back of the hand, resulting in a distal radial fracture with anterior displacement — a reversed Colles' fracture.

(2) Exclude median nerve damage (see page 210).

MANAGEMENT

(1) Reduce the fracture under a Bier's block, axillary block or general anaesthetic according to departmental policy.

(2) Reduction and immobilisation are achieved as follows:

  (i)   Disimpact the fracture by firm traction to the forearm in supination with an assistant providing countertraction to the upper arm.

  (ii) Apply pressure with the heel of the hand to reduce the distal fragment dorsally.

    (iii) Plaster the arm in full supination and dorsiflexion, e.g. with the wrist extended.

    (iv) As the reduction is difficult to hold, a long arm plaster is needed with the elbow at a right angle:
        (a) Mould an anterior slab around the radius with a slot cut for the thumb;
        (b) Extend the plaster above elbow.

    (v) Take a check x-ray to assess the adequacy of reduction before terminating the anaesthetic.
        (a) If reduction fails, internal fixation may be necessary.

(3) Give the patient a sling and analgesics and review in the next fracture clinic.

BARTON'S FRACTURE-DISLOCATION

DIAGNOSIS

This is an intra-articular fracture-dislocation of the distal radius, with the fracture line entering the wrist joint (not parallel to it as in a Smith's fracture) and the hand displaced anteriorly.

MANAGEMENT

Refer the patient immediately to the orthopaedic team as this injury is unstable and open reduction with internal fixation is required.

DISTAL RADIAL FRACTURES IN CHILDREN

DIAGNOSIS

(1) There is marked local tenderness, sometimes with deformity.
(2) X-ray will reveal a greenstick fracture that may or may not be angulated, or a slipped radial epiphysis with dorsal displacement like a Colles' fracture, most commonly in adolescents.

MANAGEMENT

(1) Refer all angulated greenstick fractures and slipped radial epiphyses to the orthopaedic team.

(2) Otherwise for a minimally buckled cortex, that may be difficult to even see on an x-ray, place the arm in a Colles'-type plaster backslab and refer the patient to the next fracture clinic.

FRACTURES OF THE SCAPHOID

DIAGNOSIS

(1) A fall on to the outstretched hand causes this common fracture, which must be considered in any patient presenting with a 'sprained wrist', particularly after a sporting injury.

(2) There is pain on dorsiflexion or ulnar deviation of the wrist and applying pressure along the thumb metacarpal. Localised tenderness in the anatomical 'snuff box' between extensor pollicis longus and abductor pollicis longus and weakness of pinch grip are seen.

(3) The x-ray request should ask specifically for scaphoid views as well as for AP and lateral wrist views.

MANAGEMENT

(1) If the x-rays are normal and pain or tenderness are minor, place the wrist in a removable splint or a double elasticated stockinette (Tubigrip) bandage and a high-arm sling.

    (i)   All x-rays must then be viewed by a senior doctor within 3 days to avoid missing an unrecognised injury.

    (ii)   Review the patient within 10 days and repeat the x-ray if the pain persists.

(2) Otherwise, if a fracture is confirmed on x-ray, or there is marked pain and tenderness particularly on moving the thumb or wrist, place the forearm in a scaphoid plaster.

(3) The scaphoid plaster (see Fig. 9):

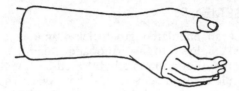

Fig. 9. The scaphoid plaster. This extends from the angle of the elbow to the metacarpal heads, and around the base of the thumb to below the interphalangeal joint.

  (i)   This extends from the angle of the elbow to the metacarpal heads including the base of the thumb to below the interphalangeal joint.

  (ii)   The wrist should be fully pronated, radially deviated, partially dorsiflexed and the thumb held in midabduction.

(4) Give the patient a high-arm sling and refer to the next fracture clinic:

  (i)   The plaster may then be reviewed and replaced if it was badly applied by the accident doctor.

  (ii)   It also allows the orthopaedic team to exclude other missed injuries such as a Bennett's fracture of the base of the thumb metacarpal, a radial styloid fracture or scapholunate dissociation.

DISLOCATIONS OF THE CARPUS

DIAGNOSIS

(1) Dislocations of the carpus are uncommon, and are caused by a fall on the outstretched hand. Two important types are seen:

  (i)   *Dislocation of the lunate.* The distal carpal bones and hand maintain their normal alignment with the radius, but the lunate is squeezed out anteriorly, like a pip.

  (ii)   *Perilunate dislocation of the carpus.* The lunate maintains its alignment with the radius, but the distal carpal bones and the hand are driven dorsally. A displaced fracture through the scaphoid may be present.

(2) The median nerve may be compressed in dislocation of the lunate, causing loss of sensation in the radial three-and-a-half digits and weakness of abductor pollicis.

(3) X-rays are easily misinterpreted as normal in lunate dislocation but:

   (i)   On the AP view the normal curved joint space between the distal radius and the scaphoid and lunate is disrupted and the lunate looks triangular instead of quadrilateral;

   (ii) On the lateral view, the dislocated lunate lies anteriorly in the shape of the letter 'C'.

MANAGEMENT

Refer all cases immediately to the orthopaedic team, particularly if median nerve compression is found.

FRACTURES OF THE OTHER CARPAL BONES

DIAGNOSIS

(1) These fractures are rare, and include fractures of the capitate, flake fracture of the triquetrum, hook of hamate fracture and pisiform fracture.

(2) There is localised tenderness from direct trauma, sometimes with an associated ulnar nerve palsy affecting the deep branch that supplies most of the intrinsic hand muscles.

(3) A common problem on x-ray is remembering the names of the eight carpal bones! Use the mnemonic 'Hamlet Came To Town Shouting Loudly To Polonius', corresponding to: hamate, capitate, trapezoid, trapezium, scaphoid, lunate, triquetral, pisiform (see Fig. 10).

MANAGEMENT

Place all these fractures in a scaphoid plaster and refer to the next fracture clinic.

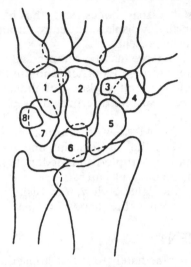

Fig. 10. The eight carpal bones. 1 Hamate. 2 Capitate. 3 Trapezoid.
4 Trapezium. 5 Scaphoid. 6 Lunate. 7 Triquetral. 8 Pisiform.

FRACTURES OF THE THUMB METACARPAL

DIAGNOSIS

(1) Injury usually results from forced thumb abduction, causing localised pain and tenderness.

(2) X-ray is always required and will distinguish stable from unstable injuries:

   (i)   Stable injuries include transverse shaft and greenstick fractures.

   (ii)   Unstable injuries include oblique shaft and comminuted fractures, and the fracture-dislocation of the base of the thumb (Bennett's fracture).

   (iii) A Bennett's fracture is an oblique fracture through the base of the thumb metacarpal involving the joint with the trapezium, with subluxation of the rest of the thumb radially:

       (a) look for swelling of the thenar eminence sometimes with local palmar bruising;

(b) make sure x-rays include the base of the thumb to avoid missing this injury.

MANAGEMENT

(1) Refer unstable fractures (including Bennett's) to the orthopaedic team for possible open reduction and internal fixation.

(2) Otherwise, for stable fractures place the hand in a scaphoid plaster and refer the patient to the next fracture clinic.

DISLOCATION OF THE THUMB METACARPAL

DIAGNOSIS

(1) This may occur in motorcycle, skiing and soccer accidents, from forced thumb abduction or hyperextension.

(2) X-ray is needed to exclude an associated fracture.

MANAGEMENT

(1) Reduce under a general anaesthetic, a local Bier's block or with an intravenous analgesic and sedative combination:

    (i)   Apply traction to the thumb with pressure over the metacarpal head. After the manipulation, repeat the x-ray to confirm the reduction.

    (ii)   Place the forearm in a scaphoid plaster with plenty of cotton-wool padding and refer the patient to the next fracture clinic.

(2) If the reduction fails, refer the patient immediately to the orthopaedic team. The metacarpal head may have 'button holed' through the joint capsule between tendons and will require open reduction.

RUPTURE OF THE ULNAR COLLATERAL LIGAMENT

DIAGNOSIS

(1) This condition ('gamekeeper's thumb' which actually used to refer to a chronic lesion) is caused by forced thumb abduction, typically in a skiing accident.

(2) It is often missed and must be suspected whenever pain and swelling are seen around the metacarpophalangeal (MCP) joint of the thumb after an abduction injury.

(3) Look for tenderness over the ulnar aspect of the MCP joint. Test for laxity of the ulnar collateral ligament by applying an abduction stress to the proximal phalanx, although pain may prevent this.

(4) X-ray may show an avulsion fracture off the proximal phalanx or a degree of MCP joint subluxation.

MANAGEMENT

Refer all cases immediately to the orthopaedic team as permanent disability may follow missed or untreated ruptures.

FRACTURES OF THE OTHER METACARPALS

DIAGNOSIS

(1) These are caused by direct trauma and may be multiple. The classical, isolated, little-finger metacarpal neck fracture or boxer's fracture is due to punching a hard object.

(2) All cases should be x-rayed and examined, particularly for any residual rotational deformity. On flexing the fingers into the palm, the fingertips should point to the scaphoid. If not, a rotational deformity of that finger exists.

MANAGEMENT

(1) Refer multiple fractures, rotated fractures, compound fractures and fractures associated with marked soft-tissue swelling from crushing immediately to the orthopaedic team.

(2) Otherwise, for undisplaced, isolated fractures give the patient a high-arm sling, an analgesic such as paraceta-

mol 500 mg and codeine phosphate 8 mg (co-codamol) and either a padded crêpe bandage or a plaster-of-Paris volar slab with the hand in the 'position of safe splintage'.

(3) Position of safe splintage:

   (i)   The volar slab extends over the flexor aspect of the forearm, on to the palm of the hand to the fingertips well padded with cotton-wool.

   (ii)   The wrist is held extended, the MCP joints flexed, the interphalangeal joints extended and the thumb abducted by the slab, which is kept in place with a cotton bandage.

   (iii)   Instruct the patient to keep the hand elevated.

   (iv)   Refer all patients to the next fracture clinic.

(4) For the isolated, little-finger knuckle injury:

   (i)   If there is over 45° angulation, refer the patient immediately to the orthopaedic team.

   (ii)   Otherwise, many different methods of reduction have been tried, but simple neighbour-strapping of the little finger, a padded crêpe bandage, a sling and analgesia is as effective as any.

   (iii)   Remember that if the knuckle struck a tooth and the skin was broken, this is potentially a very serious injury that may involve underlying tendons or even penetrate the joint capsule:

      (a) Explore the wound in the neutral position and with the fist clenched. If there is any suggestion of penetration into the joint space or tendon, refer the patient immediately to the orthopaedic team for intravenous antibiotics and full surgical exploration and debridement.

      (b) Otherwise, take a wound swab for bacterial culture and irrigate the wound with normal saline. Give the patient co-amoxiclav 500/125 (amoxycillin 500 mg, clavulanic acid 125 mg) one tablet t.d.s. for 5 days and tetanus prophylaxis.

      (c) Review the wound within 24 h.

FRACTURES OF THE PROXIMAL AND MIDDLE PHALANGES

DIAGNOSIS

(1) Similar mechanisms of injury and rules of management apply as described previously for metacarpal fractures.
(2) All cases must be examined for rotational deformity; check that on flexing the fingers into the palm, the tips point to the scaphoid.
(3) All injuries should be x-rayed to look for fractures, dislocations, subluxations and radio-opaque foreign bodies.

MANAGEMENT

(1) Refer all multiple, compound, angulated or rotated fractures, and those associated with marked soft-tissue damage or involving a joint surface to the orthopaedic team.
(2) Otherwise, neighbour-strap the finger, give the patient a high-arm sling to prevent oedema and an analgesic such as paracetamol 500 mg and codeine phosphate 8 mg (co-codamol). Refer to the next fracture clinic.

FRACTURES OF THE DISTAL PHALANGES

DIAGNOSIS

(1) These fractures are usually caused by a crushing injury resulting in a comminuted fracture of the bone.
(2) The main problem is the associated soft-tissue injury to the nail and pulp space.

MANAGEMENT

(1) Provide adequate protection by using a plastic mallet-finger splint, elevate the hand and give analgesics.
(2) *Nail injuries*:
    (i)   If the nail is avulsed, cover the exposed bed with soft paraffin gauze, give tetanus prophylaxis and flucloxacillin 500 mg orally q.d.s. for 5 days.

(ii)   If the nail is partially avulsed from the base, remove it using a ring block, in order to exclude an underlying nail-bed injury. Debride the area, remove any dirt then replace the nail as a splint to the nail matrix and a dressing to the nail-bed.

(iii) The nail-bed may need repositioning with one or two fine sutures inserted into the sides of the tip of the finger (not into the nail-bed). Dress the area, give tetanus prophylaxis and antibiotics as above, and elevate the hand in a high-arm sling.

(3) *Subungual haematoma*. Relieve this is by trephining the nail with a red-hot paper clip to release the blood under tension. If there is an associated fracture give flucloxacillin 500 mg orally q.d.s. for 5 days.

DISLOCATION OF THE PHALANGES

DIAGNOSIS AND MANAGEMENT

(1) Dislocations of the phalanges result from hyperextension injuries and must be x-rayed to exclude an associated fracture. They almost always displace dorsally, or to one side.

(2) They may be reduced under a ring block by traction applied to the finger, followed by a repeat x-ray to confirm adequate reduction.

(3) Immobilise by neighbour-strapping, and encourage active finger movements. Refer the patient to the next fracture clinic.

(4) Complications include:
   (i)   Rupture of the middle slip of the extensor tendon following proximal interphalangeal joint dislocation (see below).

   (ii)   Avulsion of the volar plate or rupture of one or both collateral ligaments. Accompanying small avulsion flake fractures may be seen on x-ray.

   (iii) Button-holing of the head of the phalanx through the volar plate necessitating open reduction.

EXTENSOR TENDON INJURIES IN THE HAND

DIAGNOSIS

(1) Injury can occur from a direct laceration, or by avulsion of the middle slip of the extensor tendon that inserts on to the middle phalanx or of the distal slip that inserts on to the distal phalanx.

(2) Demonstration of an extensor tendon injury:
- (i) Avulsion of the distal insertion causes a 'mallet-finger' deformity. The patient is unable to extend the distal interphalangeal joint with the middle phalanx being held.
- (ii) Avulsion of the middle slip that inserts on to the middle phalanx may be missed:
  - (a) Initially the proximal interphalangeal joint may be extended by the two lateral bands, but as they displace volarwards they then act as flexors;
  - (b) Finally the proximal interphalangeal joint becomes flexed and the distal interphalangeal joint hyperextended resulting in the boutonnière deformity.

(3) X-ray may show an associated flake fracture of avulsed bone.

MANAGEMENT

(1) Refer a lacerated tendon or middle slip avulsion immediately to the orthopaedic team.

(2) Manage a mallet-finger deformity in a plastic mallet-finger extension splint for 6 weeks and refer the patient to the fracture clinic.
- (i) If more than one-third of the articular surface of the distal phalanx has been avulsed, refer the patient immediately to the orthopaedic team for consideration of open reduction and internal fixation.

FLEXOR TENDON INJURIES IN THE HAND

DIAGNOSIS

(1) These injuries occur from direct laceration or blunt injury.
(2) Testing for a flexor tendon injury:
  (i)   Flexor digitorum profundus causes flexion at the distal interphalangeal joint.
  (ii)   Flexor digitorum superficialis causes flexion of the finger at the proximal interphalangeal joint, whilst the neighbouring fingers are held extended.
  (iii) A partial tendon division may be suspected by pain or reduced function against resistance.

MANAGEMENT

Give tetanus prophylaxis for any penetrating wounds. Refer all suspected flexor tendon injuries directly to the orthopaedic team.

DIGITAL NERVE INJURIES

DIAGNOSIS

(1) It is mandatory to test for digital nerve function before using any local anaesthetic blocks!
(2) Sensory loss, paraesthesiae or dryness of the skin from absent sweating, demonstrated along either side of a digit, indicate digital nerve injury.

MANAGEMENT

(1) Refer nerve injuries proximal to the proximal interphalangeal joint, to the ulnar border of the little finger, the radial border of the index finger and to the thumb immediately to the orthopaedic team.
(2) Injuries distal to the proximal interphalangeal joint rarely justify repair unless local departmental policy dictates otherwise.

FINGER TIP INJURIES

MANAGEMENT

(1) Clean and debride injuries of the distal half-centimetre that do not involve the terminal phalanx and leave to granulate under a soft paraffin-gauze dressing changed after 2 days.
(2) Give tetanus prophylaxis.
(3) Refer injuries involving substantial soft-tissue loss, distal phalanx exposure or degloving directly to the orthopaedic team.

CERVICAL SPINE INJURIES

See page 142.

THORACIC AND LUMBAR SPINE INJURIES

See page 162.

PELVIC INJURIES

See page 160.

INJURIES TO THE HIP AND UPPER FEMUR

DISLOCATION OF THE HIP

DIAGNOSIS

(1) Dislocation of the hip occurs in violent trauma such as a traffic accident, a fall from a height or sometimes a direct fall on to the hip.

(2) The commonest direction to dislocate is posteriorly (85%), as when the knee strikes the dashboard of a car. Other associated injuries from this type of accident are a fractured femoral shaft and a fractured patella.

(3) Less common are the central dislocation, fracturing through the acetabulum, or the rare anterior dislocation.

(4) In posterior dislocation the hip is held slightly flexed, adducted and internally rotated, whereas in an anterior dislocation the hip is abducted and externally rotated.

(5) Check for sciatic nerve damage in posterior dislocation of the hip, particularly if an acetabular rim fracture is present. Assess dorsiflexion (L5) and plantar flexion (S1) of the foot, and sensation over the medial side of the foot (L5) and the lateral border of the foot (S1).

MANAGEMENT

(1) Commence an intravenous infusion of normal saline and send blood for FBC, U&E, blood sugar and G&S.

(2) Give morphine 2.5–5 mg i.v. and an antiemetic such as metoclopramide 10 mg i.v.

(3) X-ray the pelvis, hip and the shaft of the femur.

(4) Refer all cases to the orthopaedic team.

FRACTURES OF THE NECK OF FEMUR

DIAGNOSIS

(1) These fractures are most common in elderly women following a fall, and may be divided into two groups:
   (i) *Intracapsular*: subcapital and transcervical;
   (ii) *Extracapsular*: intertrochanteric and pertro-chanteric.

(2) Typically after a fall, the patient is unable to weight-bear and the leg is shortened and externally rotated.

(3) Occasionally, if the fracture impacts, the patient may be able to walk, but examination reveals localised tenderness and pain on rotating the hip.

(4) X-rays must always include the pelvis, as well as AP and lateral views of the hip. A CXR is helpful as a preoperative aid for the anaesthetist.

(i)   If no femoral neck fracture is seen, look carefully for a fractured pubic ramus, as this also presents with hip pain and a limp.

MANAGEMENT

(1) Send blood for FBC, U&E, blood sugar, G&S and record an ECG.
(2) Refer the patient to the orthopaedic team, after giving intravenous analgesia titrated to response.

FRACTURES OF THE SHAFT OF FEMUR

DIAGNOSIS

(1) These fractures are due to considerable violence, as in a traffic accident, crushing injury or fall from a height.
(2) They may be associated with a hip dislocation, pelvic fracture or fracture of the patella, and cause concealed haemorrhage of 1–2 litres in a closed injury (more if compound).
(3) Rarely there is damage to the femoral vessels or sciatic nerve (under 3%).
(4) Always x-ray the pelvis, hip and knee, as well as the shaft of femur, to avoid missing these other injuries.

MANAGEMENT

(1) Give the patient oxygen, insert a large-bore intravenous cannula, and send blood for FBC, U&E and blood sugar. Cross-match 4 units of blood and commence an infusion of normal saline or polygeline (Haemaccel).
(2) Perform a femoral nerve block to relieve the pain:
   (i)   Palpate the femoral artery and insert a 21-gauge needle with syringe perpendicular to the skin, lateral to the artery and just below the inguinal ligament.
   (ii)   If paraesthesia is elicited down the leg indicating proximity of the needle to the nerve, withdraw slightly, aspirate to exclude vessel puncture and in

adults inject 10 ml of 0.5% bupivacaine i.e. 50 mg (maximum safe dosage is 2 mg/kg).

   (iii)   Alternatively, a characteristic loss of resistance may be felt as the needle passes through the fascia lata then fascia iliaca:

        (a) aspirate to exclude vessel puncture;

        (b) inject 10 ml of 0.5% bupivacaine fanwise moving out up to 3 cm lateral to the artery.

(3) If pain persists despite a femoral nerve block, give morphine 2.5–5 mg i.v. and an antiemetic such as metoclopramide 10 mg i.v.

(4) Apply traction as quickly as possible to reduce the pain and blood loss, and to facilitate movement of the patient during x-ray (x-rays should be done after the splint is in place).

(5) Use a commercially available Donway Traction Splint.

(6) Alternatively, use a traditional skin traction device such as the Thomas splint:

   (i)   Select the size of Thomas splint by measuring the oblique circumference around the top of the thigh and adding 4 cm, and the distance from the greater trochanter to the heel adding 20 cm, to give the length.

   (ii) Shave the lateral and medial sides of the thigh and lower leg and spray with tincture of benzoin.

   (iii) Maintain firm traction on the leg as the adhesive strapping of the skin traction set is applied to the whole length of the leg, ensuring the malleoli are protected by the foam.

   (iv) Secure the adhesive strapping with crêpe bandages.

   (v)   Slip a double layer of circular elasticated stockinette (Tubigrip) over the splint; then slide the splint over the leg, which rests on the stockinette base.

   (vi) Protect the groin area with cotton-wool padding, and pad underneath the fracture and knee as well.

   (vii) Tie the skin traction to the end of the splint and tighten it by twisting four wooden spatulae inserted between the ropes as a Chinese windlass.

(viii) Finally, secure the leg on the splint with further crêpe bandages, and raise the leg by placing a pillow under the foot.
(ix) Check the pulse in the foot is still present.
(7) Refer the patient to the orthopaedic team.

INJURIES TO THE LOWER FEMUR, KNEE AND UPPER TIBIA

SUPRACONDYLAR AND CONDYLAR FRACTURES OF THE FEMUR

DIAGNOSIS

(1) These injuries are caused by direct trauma or a fall in an elderly person with osteoporotic bones.
(2) The popliteal artery is only rarely damaged by supracondylar fractures, although condylar fractures often cause a tense haemarthrosis.

MANAGEMENT

Give the patient analgesics and refer immediately to the orthopaedic team, for aspiration of any tense haemarthrosis and operative fixation in certain cases.

FRACTURES OF THE PATELLA AND INJURY TO THE QUADRICEPS APPARATUS

DIAGNOSIS

(1) Damage is caused by direct trauma as in a traffic accident or fall, or by indirect violence from quadriceps contraction.
(2) Remember to always examine the shaft of femur and the hip.

(3) If the quadriceps mechanism is damaged, in most cases there is inability to extend the knee associated with local pain.

(4) X-ray will demonstrate the patella fracture:
  - (i) Confusion may arise from congenital bipartite or tripartite patellae, although these are often bilateral, unlike fractures.
  - (ii) The presence of a lipohaemarthrosis causing a horizontal line fluid level on the lateral x-ray view of the knee is a helpful indicator of intra-articular fracture.

MANAGEMENT

(1) Refer a distracted or comminuted fracture, or any damage to the extensor mechanism of the knee directly to the orthopaedic team.

(2) Otherwise, if there is a stable, undisplaced fracture of the patella, place the leg in a padded plaster cylinder from the thigh to the ankle and refer the patient to the next fracture clinic.

(3) If there is a tense haemarthrosis this may be aspirated first, before applying the plaster cylinder.

(4) Aspiration of the knee:
  - (i) Use a strict aseptic technique. Clean the skin with povidone-iodine and inject 2% lignocaine 2–3 ml into the skin, subcutaneous tissue and synovium.
  - (ii) Insert a 14-gauge cannula at the midpoint of the superior portion of the patella, 1 cm lateral to the anterolateral edge.
  - (iii) Aim the cannula between the posterior surface of the patella and the intercondylar femoral notch.
  - (iv) Withdraw the needle and attach a 50 ml syringe with 3-way tap to the remaining catheter. Aspirate to dryness. Gently squeeze the suprapatellar region to 'milk' any residual fluid.
  - (v) Up to 70 ml bloodstained fluid may be removed. Look for evidence of fat globules floating on the surface of the blood to confirm an intra-articular fracture.

DISLOCATION OF THE PATELLA

DIAGNOSIS

(1) The patella commonly dislocates laterally in teenage girls and may become recurrent.

(2) Sometimes spontaneous reduction occurs and the patient then presents with a tender knee particularly along the medial border of the patella.

    (i)   A careful history and 'patella apprehension', as the patella is pushed laterally causing pain, suggest the true diagnosis.

MANAGEMENT

(1) Reduce by firm pressure with extension of the knee, pushing the patella medially under inhaled nitrous oxide with oxygen (Entonox) analgesia.

(2) Request a skyline patellar x-ray after the reduction to exclude an associated osteochondral fracture.

(3) Place the leg in a padded plaster cylinder and refer the patient to the next fracture clinic.

(4) If the dislocation is recurrent, use a pressure bandage instead of a plaster cylinder.

SOFT-TISSUE INJURIES OF THE KNEE

A careful history of the mechanism of injury and the subsequent events is crucial, as examination is often difficult in an acutely painful knee. Always lie the patient on an examination trolley and undress properly.

DIAGNOSIS

(1) A rapid swelling of the knee indicates a haemarthrosis, usually due to an anterior cruciate tear, peripheral meniscal tear or intra-articular fracture. A delayed swelling, occurring after several hours, suggests a serous effusion.

(2) Injuries may be suspected from the direction of force:

    (i)   Sideways stresses will rupture the collateral ligaments or joint capsule.

    (ii)   A twisting injury will damage one of the menisci, usually the medial.

    (iii)   Combinations may be seen. A severe lateral blow to the knee, e.g. from a car bumper, will rupture the medial collateral ligament, tear the medial meniscus and rupture the anterior cruciate ligament (O'Donoghue's triad).

(3) Examination must include:

    (i)   Palpating for the area of maximum pain;

    (ii)   Assessing the medial and lateral collateral ligaments by stressing each side with the knee slightly flexed;

    (iii)   Assessing the cruciates by attempting to move the tibia backwards (posterior cruciate) or abnormally forwards (anterior cruciate) with the knee flexed

        (a)   Beware that a posterior cruciate tear allows the head of the tibia to slip backwards, which will then move forwards into a correct position on stressing (but not into an abnormal position as in an anterior cruciate tear).

(4) Meniscal tears may result in 'locking' of the knee with inability to extend the knee fully.

(5) All patients must be x-rayed to exclude associated fractures such as:

    (i)   A tibial condyle fracture;

    (ii)   Avulsion fracture of the tibial spines in cruciate ligament tears;

    (iii)   Flake fractures of the lateral or medial femoral condyles in collateral ligament tears;

    (iv)   Avulsion of the tibial tubercle (Osgood–Schlatter's disease due to traction apophysitis most commonly in young male teenagers).

MANAGEMENT

(1) Refer the following to the orthopaedic team:

    (i)   a tense effusion including all suspected haemarthroses;

    (ii)   a 'locked' knee (sudden loss of ability to extend the knee fully);

(iii)   a suspected torn ligament;
(iv)   an associated fracture;
(v)   any penetrating wound of the knee suggested by air or foreign material in the joint on x-ray, although these may be absent.

(2) Otherwise, if there is only moderate swelling, a good range of joint movement and no ligamentous laxity:

(i)   apply a double elasticated stockinette bandage (Tubigrip) to the knee;
(ii)   give the patient anti-inflammatory analgesics such as diclofenac 50 mg orally t.d.s. or naproxen 500 mg orally b.d.;
(iii) lend the patient crutches to use until the acute symptoms settle;
(iv)   review the patient within 5 days.

Note: in patients presenting with knee pain, always examine the hip and spine as the pain may be referred, particularly in children; hence the need to undress the patient.

DISLOCATION OF THE KNEE

DIAGNOSIS AND MANAGEMENT

(1) This is a severe injury with up to 30% incidence of damage to the popliteal vessels and lateral popliteal nerve.
(2) Give the patient analgesics, check the distal pulses, x-ray and refer immediately to the orthopaedic team.

FRACTURES OF THE TIBIAL CONDYLES

DIAGNOSIS

(1) These fractures are caused by falls from a height, or severe lateral or medial stresses which in addition may rupture the knee ligaments.
(2) A tense haemarthrosis is usual and precludes further detailed examination of the knee due to pain.
(3) Always check for vascular damage by palpating the foot pulses. Check for a lateral popliteal nerve palsy by

testing for active foot dorsiflexion and eversion, and sensation over the lateral aspect of the calf.

(4) X-ray will show the tibial condyle fracture either laterally or (rarely) on the medial side although sometimes they are subtle and difficult to see.

    (i)   Look for a horizontal line fluid level in the suprapatellar pouch on the lateral view due to a lipohaemarthrosis, indicating an intra-articular fracture.

MANAGEMENT

Give the patient analgesics and refer immediately to the orthopaedic team.

INJURIES TO THE LOWER TIBIA, ANKLE AND FOOT

FRACTURES OF THE SHAFT OF THE TIBIA

DIAGNOSIS

(1) Direct trauma is responsible for most of these injuries, which are often compound. Greenstick fractures in children and stress fractures in athletes are also seen.

(2) X-rays should always include the knee and ankle, as well as the shaft of the tibia.

MANAGEMENT

(1) Compound injuries:

    (i)   Send blood for FBC, U&E and blood sugar. Cross-match 2 units of blood and commence an intravenous infusion of normal saline.

    (ii)   Give the patient morphine 2.5–5 mg i.v. with an antiemetic such as metoclopramide 10 mg i.v., restore anatomical alignment and cover the exposed area with a sterile dressing.

    (iii)   Give flucloxacillin 1 g i.v., benzylpenicillin 1 Mu (600 mg) i.v. and tetanus prophylaxis.

    (iv)   Use a temporary plastic adjustable splint or a long-leg plaster backslab for support, especially if there are other injuries to the chest or abdomen requiring more urgent care.

    (v)   Refer the patient immediately to the orthopaedic team.

(2) Refer all other tibial shaft fractures to the orthopaedic team, having given the patient analgesics and provided a suitable splint.

ISOLATED FRACTURE OF THE FIBULA

DIAGNOSIS AND MANAGEMENT

(1) This is caused by a direct blow, typically at soccer.

(2) Provided there is definitely no injury to the ankle, and no tibial fracture at another level, use:

    (i)   A firm crêpe bandage with cotton-wool padding,

    (ii)   Or a below-knee walking plaster that affords more protection.

(3) Refer the patient to the next fracture clinic.

PRETIBIAL LACERATIONS

DIAGNOSIS

These are most common in elderly patients, often from trivial trauma tearing a flap of skin.

MANAGEMENT

(1) Clean the wound and trim any obviously necrotic tissue.

(2) If there is actual skin loss or marked skin retraction preventing alignment of the skin edges, refer the patient immediately to the surgical team for early skin grafting.

(3) Otherwise, lay the flap back over the wound and hold it in place with adhesive skin-closure strips (Steristrips). Cover the wound with a single layer of paraffin-impreg-

nated gauze (Jelonet) and a cotton-wool and gauze pad (Gamgee).
(4) Then apply a firm crêpe bandage and instruct the patient to keep the leg elevated whenever possible.
(5) Review the patient after 5 days, removing the dressing but leaving the Steristrips in place.
  (i) If the skin is now obviously nonviable, refer the patient to the orthopaedic or surgical team for skin grafting.
  (ii) Otherwise, if healing is taking place, review the patient weekly or discharge to the care of the general practitioner and district nurse.

INVERSION ANKLE INJURIES

DIAGNOSIS

(1) These injuries are common following sports injuries, or trips on staircases or uneven ground.
(2) The aim is to distinguish ligament tears from bony injury, and to assess the stability of the ankle.
  (i) Immediate swelling and inability to weight-bear suggest a fracture or serious ligament tear.
  (ii) Examine for the sites of maximum pain:
    (a) over the distal fibula and lateral malleolus itself;
    (b) over the anterior talofibular portion of the lateral ligament of the ankle, over the posterior talofibular portion or the middle calcaneofibular portion;
    (c) around the medial malleolus or over the medial deltoid ligament;
    (d) over the anterior tibiofibular ligament;
    (e) over the base of the fifth metatarsal;
    (f) over the navicular;
    (g) around the calcaneus.
(3) An AP and lateral x-ray of the ankle should be requested if there is pain in the malleolar area and any of the following:[1]
  (i) bone tenderness over the posterior edge or tip of the distal 6 cm of the lateral malleolus;

     (ii)   or bone tenderness over the posterior edge or tip of the distal 6 cm of the medial malleolus;

    (iii)   or inability to weight bear (e.g. unable to take 4 steps without assistance, regardless of limping) both within the first hour of injury and in the A&E department.

(4) Additional foot x-rays should only be requested if there is pain in the midfoot and any of the following:[1]

     (i)   bone tenderness over the base of the fifth metatarsal;

    (ii)   or bone tenderness over the navicular;

    (iii)   or inability to weight bear both immediately and in the A & E department.

MANAGEMENT

(1) Refer a displaced lateral malleolar fracture, an associated medial malleolar fracture, widening or diastasis of the ankle mortice, and severe pain or swelling immediately to the orthopaedic team.

(2) Otherwise, immobilise an avulsion flake fracture of the malleolus or talus and an undisplaced lateral malleolar fracture in a below-knee plaster:

     (i)   This is applied from the metatarsal heads to below the tibial tubercle, with the ankle at a right angle (not in equinus).

    (ii)   Repeat the ankle x-ray after application of the plaster.

    (iii)   Refer the patient to the next fracture clinic, with instructions to keep the leg elevated overnight.

(3) If the patient is able to weight-bear and no fracture is seen, with minimal swelling:

     (i)   Apply a double elasticated stockinette (Tubigrip) bandage, give the patient crutches or a walking frame, and an anti-inflammatory analgesic such as diclofenac 50 mg orally t.d.s. or naproxen 500 mg orally b.d.

    (ii)   Recommend initial elevation, no weight-bearing and a cold compress (e.g. a bag of frozen peas) at home, followed by gradual mobilisation.

(iii)   Warn patients that they will not be fully fit for active sports for at least 3 weeks, however much they protest!

(iv)   Review the patient after 5–10 days and refer to physiotherapy if there is persisting disability.

OTHER ANKLE INJURIES

DIAGNOSIS

(1) Eversion injuries damaging the medial malleolus and medial deltoid ligament, hyperflexion injuries or rotational injuries tend to cause more complicated damage.

(2) Examine the ankle as before to localise the maximum area of tenderness. In addition, palpate the upper fibula for a high (Maisonneuve) fracture associated with tibiofibular diastasis and a widened ankle mortice.

(3) X-ray all patients meeting the criteria on page 243 and include the upper tibia and fibula if there is proximal tenderness.

MANAGEMENT

(1) Refer all fractures, widened ankle mortices or patients totally unable to weight-bear to the orthopaedic team.

(2) Otherwise treat as in 3(i) to 3(iv) above.

DISLOCATION OF THE ANKLE

DIAGNOSIS AND MANAGEMENT

(1) This dislocation is most commonly posterior and is clinically obvious. It must be reduced immediately to prevent ischaemic pressure necrosis of skin stretched across the malleolus.

(2) Give the patient morphine 5 mg i.v. and metoclopramide 10 mg i.v.

(i)   Then give midazolam 2.5–5 mg i.v. in a monitored area with resuscitation equipment available.

(ii) Reduce the ankle dislocation by steady traction on the heel, gently dorsiflexing the foot.

(iii)   After the reduction, place the lower leg in a plastic splint or padded backslab before sending the patient for post-reduction x-ray.

(3) Refer the patient immediately to the orthopaedic team.

FRACTURES AND DISLOCATION OF THE TALUS

DIAGNOSIS

(1) The talus articulates in three joints: the ankle joint with the tibia and fibula, the subtalar joint with the calcaneus and the midtarsal joint with the navicular (along with the calcaneus and cuboid).

(2) It is injured by falls from a height or sudden violence to the foot, as from the pedal of a car being forced upwards in a traffic accident.

(3) There is pain and swelling, and x-ray is needed to define the injuries.

MANAGEMENT

(1) Refer all fractures including the osteochondral dome fracture immediately to the orthopaedic team.

(2) The only exception is an avulsion flake fracture of the neck of the talus from a ligamentous or capsular insertion, which may be treated in a below-knee plaster and referred to the next fracture clinic.

(3) Complications of talar injuries include avascular necrosis and persistent pain and disability from osteoarthrosis, particularly if the injury is missed.

(4) Occasionally the talus can dislocate completely and lie laterally in front of the ankle joint, requiring urgent manipulation to avoid overlying skin necrosis, similar to the dislocated ankle.

FRACTURES OF THE CALCANEUS

DIAGNOSIS

(1) These are usually due to a fall from a height, and are bilateral in 20%.

(2) Falls from a height are associated with a characteristic pattern of injuries that includes fractures to:
  (i)   calcaneus;
  (ii)   ankle;
  (iii) tibial plateau;
  (iv)   femoral head or hip;
  (v)   thoracolumbar vertebra;
  (vi)   atlas and base of the skull.
  Each of these must be specifically looked for in turn and any tender areas x-rayed.
(3) The heel tends to flatten following a calcaneal fracture, and is locally tender with bruising spreading onto the sole and up the calf.
(4) Request an AP and lateral ankle x-ray with an additional tangential (axial) calcaneal view to avoid missing the fracture.
(5) A CT scan may be necessary to demonstrate involvement of the subtalar joint.

MANAGEMENT

Refer all fractures to the orthopaedic team. Keep the patient's foot elevated and give an analgesic.

RUPTURE OF THE TENDO ACHILLIS

DIAGNOSIS

(1) This injury is most common in middle-aged men following abrupt muscular activity. There is pain and weakness of plantar flexion, although some is still possible by the long toe flexors; however, the patient is unable to stand on tiptoe.
(2) A palpable gap in the tendon may be felt although this rapidly fills with blood.
(3) The 'calf squeeze' test shows reduced or absent foot plantar flexion compared to the uninjured side, when the relaxed calf is gently squeezed with the patient kneeling on a chair with the feet hanging free.

MANAGEMENT

Give the patient analgesics and refer to the orthopaedic team for operative repair or conservative treatment.

MIDTARSAL DISLOCATIONS

DIAGNOSIS

(1) These follow a twisting injury to the forefoot causing pain and swelling around the talonavicular and calcaneocuboid midtarsal joint.
(2) X-ray shows disruption of the midtarsal joint, often associated with fractures of the navicular, cuboid, talus or calcaneus. These may merely be avulsion flake fractures.

MANAGEMENT

Give the patient analgesics, elevate the foot and refer to the orthopaedic team.

METATARSAL INJURIES AND TARSOMETATARSAL DISLOCATIONS

DIAGNOSIS

(1) These are caused by direct trauma, crushing or twisting.
(2) A transverse avulsion fracture of the base of the fifth metatarsal is seen following ankle inversion, at the site of insertion of peroneus brevis.
(3) A stress fracture may occur, usually in the neck of the second metatarsal known as the 'march fracture'.
(4) Tarsometatarsal dislocation is uncommon and may be multiple, resulting in widening of the gap between the base of the hallux and second metatarsal with lateral shift of the remaining metatarsals.
  (i) It is often missed as the significance of the foot swelling is not appreciated and interpretation of the x-ray is difficult.
  (ii) Circulatory impairment in the forefoot must be excluded.

MANAGEMENT

(1) Refer all compound, displaced or multiple fractures, tarsometatarsal dislocations, fractures of the first metatarsal and injuries associated with considerable crushing or oedema immediately to the orthopaedic team.
(2) Treat an avulsion fracture of the base of the fifth metatarsal as for an ankle sprain, and a 'march fracture' in a support bandage, or rarely a below-knee plaster if the pain is severe.

FRACTURES OF THE PHALANGES OF THE FOOT

DIAGNOSIS AND MANAGEMENT

(1) These fractures are usually caused by a direct blow.
(2) Clean all the wounds and release any subungual haematoma by trephining.
(3) Otherwise, give an analgesic and a support bandage, having neighbour-strapped the damaged toe.
(4) If the pain is severe, particularly with injury to the great toe, use a below-knee plaster with a toe platform extension.
(5) Refer all patients to the next fracture clinic.

SOFT-TISSUE INJURIES

The so-called 'minor injury' is of major importance to the patient and may lead to serious problems if incorrectly managed. Therefore adopt a consistent, careful approach to every patient presenting with a soft-tissue injury.

GENERAL MANAGEMENT OF A SOFT-TISSUE INJURY

(1) *Assessment.*
    (i)   Obtain a history of:
        (a) the nature of the injury, and when and where it was sustained;

(b) current medical conditions and drug therapy;
(c) antibiotic allergy and tetanus immune status;
(d) the possibility of a foreign body, wound contamination and damage to deeper structures;
(e) any crushing injury.

(ii) Examine nerves and tendons for evidence of damage, before infiltrating with local anaesthetic.

(iii) If a radio-opaque foreign body (metal or glass) is suspected, send the patient for x-rays before exploring the wound. Inform the radiographer of the nature of the foreign body.

(2) *Cleaning.*

(i) After scrubbing-up and wearing sterile gloves, remove all the dirt and debris from around the edges of the wound using normal saline or a disinfectant, e.g. chlorhexidine or cetrimide, by swabbing and gentle rubbing.

(ii) Remove adjacent hair for at least 5 mm, but never shave the eyebrows or eyelashes.

(3) *Local anaesthetic infiltration.*

(i) The patient should always be lying down.

(ii) Use 1% lignocaine infiltrated along the edge of the wound with a 25-gauge orange needle.

(iii) Ring block.
Use a ring block with plain 2% lignocaine without adrenaline for wounds around the nail, fingertip and distal finger.

(a) A ring block is contraindicated in patients with peripheral vascular disease, Raynaud's phenomenon and local sepsis at the base of the finger.

(b) Do not use a tourniquet due to the risk of creating high pressures locally and occluding the digital vessels. First clean the base of the finger with antiseptic.

(c) Insert a 25-gauge orange needle into the side of the base of the finger, and angle at 45° from the vertical injecting up to 1 ml of 2% lignocaine (without adrenaline) into the lateral palmar aspect of the finger.

      (d) Remove the needle until subcutaneous, and rotate until it is pointing to the extensor surface of the finger; inject 0.5 ml into the lateral extensor aspect of the finger.

      (e) Perform the same procedure on the other side of the finger.

      (f) Allow at least 5–10 min for the block to take effect.

(iv)   The maximum safe dosage of lignocaine is 3 mg/kg. A 1% solution contains 10 mg/ml. Therefore:

      (a) 20 ml of 1% solution containing 200 mg lignocaine or

      (b) 10 ml of 2% solution containing 200 mg lignocaine are the maximum safe amounts allowed in a 67-kg patient.

(v)   Signs of lignocaine toxicity include:

      (a) perioral tingling, a metallic taste, restlessness, dizziness and slurred speech;

      (b) convulsions and coma;

      (c) bradycardia, hypotension and circulatory collapse.

Treat convulsions with intravenous diazepam, and circulatory collapse by commencing cardiopulmonary resuscitation (see page 2).

(4) *Exploration, irrigation, debridement and haemostasis.*

   (i)   Look carefully for evidence of foreign bodies, and severed tendons, vessels or nerves within the wound. Seek immediate senior help if the latter are found.

  (ii)   A 20-ml syringe filled with saline and fitted with a 23-gauge blue needle provides a useful high-pressure jet to irrigate the wound.

 (iii) Excise any dead or contaminated tissue and remove local dirt on the skin by rubbing gently.

      (a) It is particularly important to remove all ingrained gravel and grit to avoid permanent tattooing of the skin. A general anaesthetic may be required.

  (iv) Achieve haemostasis by local pressure. Avoid the use of mosquito forceps to clamp a bleeding area which may cause further local tissue damage.

(5) *Suture*.
- (i)   The aim is to appose the edges of the wound without tension using interrupted sutures, starting in the middle of the wound and halving the remaining distance each time.
  - (a)   Use an absorbable suture for deeper wounds such as chromic catgut or polyglactin to close the deep space first, with the knot buried at the depth of the wound.
- (ii)   The choice of material depends on local custom.
  - (a)   Traditionally silk was the most popular, although as it is braided and of animal origin it is more likely to cause microabscess formation with subsequent scarring.
  - (b)   Synthetic monofilament sutures such as polyamide (Ethilon) and polypropylene (Prolene) are now preferred, although harder to tie requiring an initial double throw and multiple knots, they elicit less of a foreign-body reaction.
- (iii)   Use the smallest practicable suture size.
  - (a)   Limb laceration: Use 4/0 synthetic monofilament sutures removed at 7–10 days.
  - (b)   Scalp: Use 2/0 or 3/0 synthetic monofilament sutures removed at 7 days.
  - (c)   Face: Use 5/0 or 6/0 synthetic monofilament sutures removed at 4 days.
- (iv)   Cover the wound with a nonadherent dressing and advise the patient to keep the area dry for at least 3 days.
- (v)   Give an appointment for removal of sutures in the department or with the general practitioner.
- (vi)   Make a record in the notes of the size and nature of the wound, the deep structures involved and the number of sutures used to close it.

(6) *Tetanus prophylaxis*.
- (i)   Meticulous wound toilet is an essential part of tetanus prophylaxis, rather than simply relying on tetanus immunisation or antibiotics.

(ii) In the UK, routine tetanus immunisation was introduced in 1961 so the elderly are now the most likely to be nonimmune.

(iii) Virtually any wound can become contaminated, however trivial.

(iv) Treat patients according to their immune-status category A–C (see Table 7) and to the type of wound:

    (a) *Tetanus-prone wound*: any wound over 6 h old, deep, crushed or penetrating, contaminated with soil, a compound fracture, a human or animal bite, a partial- or full-thickness burn and clinical evidence of sepsis;

    (b) *Clean wound*: any wound less than 6 h old, clean, incised or superficial, e.g. does not fulfil any criteria of a tetanus-prone wound.

(v) Local pain, redness and swelling occur with tetanus toxoid and occasionally systemic reactions, even anaphylaxis. These reactions are much less common with human tetanus immunoglobulin.

Table 7. Tetanus prophylaxis

Immune status category	Treatment	
	Tetanus-prone wound	*Clean wound*
A. Complete course of toxoid[1] or a booster[2] in last 10 years	Nothing	Nothing
B. Complete course of toxoid or a booster over 10 years ago	Toxoid booster HTIG[3]	Toxoid booster
C. Never completed a course or state of immunity unknown	Complete course of toxoid HTIG	Complete course of toxoid

[1] A complete course of toxoid is a total of three injections of 0.5 ml adsorbed tetanus toxoid i.m. given on day 1, at 4 weeks and at 2 months.

[2] A booster is a subsequent injection of 0.5 ml adsorbed tetanus toxoid i.m.

[3] HTIG is 250 U of human tetanus immunoglobulin in 1 ml given i.m. at a different site to the toxoid.

(vi) Tetanus itself is rare with around 20 cases reported annually in the UK:

   (a) Incubation time from injury to first symptoms ranges from 4 to 21 days, usually about 7.

   (b) The commonest symptoms are jaw stiffness (trismus), dysphagia, abdominal and back pain. Hypertonia is found on examination.

   (c) Localised or generalised painful spasms follow within 24–72 h, becoming more severe and prolonged from minimal stimuli.

   (d) Death may occur from laryngospasm, respiratory failure or autonomic dysfunction, therefore immediate admission to intensive care is mandatory.

(7) *Antibiotics*.

Antibiotics should not be used indiscriminately and are secondary to thorough surgical toilet in preventing infection. They are reserved for:

(i) Cellulitis:

   (a) This is usually due to a beta-haemolytic streptococcus or occasionally *Staphylococcus aureus*. Always send a swab first.

   (b) Use penicillin V 500 mg orally q.d.s. or flucloxacillin 500 mg orally q.d.s. for 1 week.

(ii) Dirty, contaminated wound:

   (a) Use amoxycillin 500 mg orally t.d.s. for 1 week.

   (b) If the wound involves bone or tendon, add flucloxacillin 500 mg orally q.d.s.

   (c) For patients allergic to penicillin, use erythromycin 500 mg orally q.d.s.

(iii) Bites:

   (a) These are best cleaned with 10% povidone-iodine. They should not be sutured except on the face.

   (b) Tetanus prophylaxis is always needed.

   (c) Prescribe according to the origin of the bite:
Human: co-amoxiclav 500/125 (amoxycillin 500 mg and clavulanic acid 125 mg) one tablet orally t.d.s. for 5 days. If penicillin sensitive

use doxycycline, or use erythromycin if pregnant, nursing or in children.

Cat: amoxicillin 500 mg orally t.d.s. for 3 days.

Dog: treat as above for cat. Consider rabies prophylaxis if the patient was bitten abroad. Discuss this with experts at the local infectious disease hospital, or contact the Communicable Disease Surveillance Centre in London (telephone 0181 200 6868).

(iv) Compound fractures:
  (a) Give flucloxacillin 1 g i.v. and benzylpenicillin 1 Mu (600 mg) i.v.
  (b) Remember tetanus prophylaxis.

CRUSH INJURIES

DIAGNOSIS

(1) Crush injuries may be caused by a roller or wringer injury, a direct blow or a vehicle wheel passing over a limb.

(2) Severe soft-tissue injury can occur with little apparent initial evidence.

(3) Test for tendon, nerve or vessel damage. Note any loss of blanching of the skin on digital pressure indicating shearing of capillaries, which may subsequently lead to extensive tissue necrosis.

(4) Always consider the possibility of a compartment syndrome if there is severe ischaemic pain particularly on passive stretching of muscles, associated with paraesthesiae and loss of motor and sensory nerve function:

  (i) Apart from crush injuries, other causes of a compartment syndrome include external compression from a tight plaster, fractures, constricting burns, bleeding, vigorous exercise and prolonged local pressure in coma, e.g. following acute poisoning.

  (ii) The entire area within the closed fascial compartment feels tense.

(iii)   However, arterial pulses and even skin perfusion may initially remain deceptively normal.

(5) X-ray is required to exclude underlying fractures.

MANAGEMENT

(1) Refer all crush injuries of a limb, hand or foot to the orthopaedic team for elevation, treatment of shock, possible fasciotomy and occasionally amputation.

(2) Otherwise, in isolated finger or toe injuries, clean and debride the wound without suturing, elevate the limb and give the patient analgesics. Review within 3 days for consideration of delayed primary suture.

PUNCTURE INJURIES

DIAGNOSIS

(1) This type of injury is caused by treading on a nail or pin, penetration of a sewing-machine needle, or through industrial accidents including those involving the high-pressure gun for grease, paint, water or oil.

(2) 'Sharps injury' within a hospital is covered on page 116.

MANAGEMENT

(1) Refer all high-pressure gun injuries immediately to the orthopaedic team, even if no apparent damage is seen initially.

(2) Otherwise clean the wound with antiseptic, give tetanus prophylaxis and consider the need for antibiotics. A rusty nail injury to the foot requires co-amoxiclav 500/125 (amoxycillin 500 mg and clavulanic acid 125 mg) one tablet orally t.d.s. for 5 days.

(3) Instruct the patient to return immediately if signs of infection or gross oedema supervene.

HAND INFECTIONS

(1) *Paronychia*:
   (i)   This is pus formation adjacent to the nail, with throbbing pain.

(ii)   Make a longitudinal incision parallel to the nail edge to release the pus, using a ring-block anaesthetic (see page 250). Mop out the cavity with pledgets of cotton-wool.

(iii) Dress the finger with paraffin-impregnated gauze tucked into the cavity, and apply a cotton tubular bandage (Tubegauz) without tension. Use a high-arm sling for 24 h and review the dressing after 2 days.

(2) *Pulp space infection*:

(i)   This is pus formation in the distal fat pad of the finger.

(ii) Using a ring block, make a central longitudinal incision over the middle of the abscess (take care not to cross the flexion crease of the distal inter phalangeal joint). Mop out the cavity of all pus.

(iii) Dress and review as for paronychia.

(iv) In more extensive infections with swelling approaching the distal interphalangeal joint, the flexor tendon sheath is in danger. Refer the patient directly to the orthopaedic team, after requesting an x-ray to exclude osteomyelitis.

(3) *Suppurative tenosynovitis of the flexor tendons*:

(i)   The original wound may have been forgotten, but intense pain, swelling and tenderness develop along the line of the flexor tendon, with severe pain on passive finger flexion.

(ii) Refer the patient directly to the orthopaedic team.

(4) *Deep palmar and web space infections*:

(i)   These cause pain, swelling and loss of function with localised tenderness and the development of a 'flipper' hand, from pronounced swelling of the dorsum of the hand.

(ii) Refer the patient directly to the orthopaedic team.

INGROWING TOENAILS

(1) These are common, associated with tight-fitting footwear or socks, poor foot hygiene and trimming off the corners of the nail. They usually afflict young people.

(2) Surgical treatment by wedge resection or total nailbed ablation requires skill and expertise, and is only as successful as the experience of the surgeon.

(3) Medical treatment:

    (i)   Liquid nitrogen spray cryotherapy requires special equipment that is usually not readily available.

    (ii)   An alternative is to insert a pledget of cotton-wool under the nail edge with a pair of forceps, and to cauterise the granulation tissue with a silver nitrate stick.

        (a) Advise the patient to wear loose shoes and of the importance of cutting the nail straight across in future.

        (b) Ask the patient to repeat the cotton-wool insertion and silver nitrate cautery once or twice a day at home.

        (c) This method is effective, cheap and requires no special apparatus.[2]

BACK PAIN

This is a common problem that may be considered under four headings:

(1) direct trauma;

(2) indirect trauma;

(3) nontraumatic — severe or atypical pain;

(4) nontraumatic — mild to moderate pain.

DIRECT TRAUMA

Back pain due to direct trauma is managed according to the principles in the appropriate chapter on multiple injuries (see page 162).

INDIRECT TRAUMA

DIAGNOSIS

(1) Acute, severe back pain may be precipitated by bending, lifting, straining, coughing or sneezing.

(2) There is intense muscle spasm, even complete immobility. The normal lumbar lordosis is lost, with development of a scoliosis.

(3) Examine for signs of nerve-root irritation and compression from an acute prolapsed disc:

   (i)   Diminished straight-leg raising (SLR). Remember that the ability to sit up in bed with the legs straight is equivalent to a SLR of 90° both sides.

   (ii)   Motor loss occurring in the following myotomes:

L1, L2	Hip flexion (iliopsoas)
S1	Hip extension (gluteus maximus)
L5	Knee flexion (hamstrings)
L3, L4	Knee extension (quadriceps)
L5	Ankle dorsiflexion (extensor hallucis longus)
S1	Ankle plantar flexion (calf muscles).

   (iii)   Reflex loss:

L3, L4	Knee jerk
L5, S1	Ankle jerk

   (iv)   Sensory loss occurring in the following dermatomes:

L3	Medial lower thigh and knee
L4	Medial side of calf
L5	Lateral side of calf
S1	Lateral border of the foot and sole.

(4) Examine in particular for signs of a central disc prolapse causing cauda equina compression:

   (i)   Difficulty emptying the bladder or bowels;

   (ii)   Lax anal sphincter tone;

   (iii)   Saddle area anaesthesia over dermatomes S2, S3, S4 and S5;

   (iv)   Weakness in both legs.

MANAGEMENT

(1) Refer any patient with a central disc prolapse causing cauda equina compression immediately to the orthopaedic team.

(2) Also, if the patient is completely unable to move or has signs of nerve-root compression, refer to the orthopaedic team for admission.

(3) Patients with only moderate pain and without nerve-root signs may be discharged:
   (i)   Give the patient a nonsteroidal anti-inflammatory analgesic such as diclofenac 50 mg orally t.d.s.
   (ii) Encourage a rapid return to ordinary activities within the limits of pain. Bed rest should be kept to a minimum.[3]
   (iii) Request review and follow-up by the general practitioner for back care education including posture, exercise and lifting.

NONTRAUMATIC — SEVERE OR ATYPICAL PAIN

DIAGNOSIS

(1) The causes vary according to the patient's age:
   (i)   Under 30 years:
         (a) ankylosing spondylitis;
         (b) rheumatoid arthritis;
         (c) osteomyelitis;
         (d) discitis;
         (e) extradural abscess.
   (ii) Over 30 years:
         (a) bony metastases;
         (b) myeloma;
         (c) lymphoma;
         (d) renal or pancreatic disease;
         (e) aortic aneurysm.
   (iii) Over 60 years:
         (a) as (ii) above;
         (b) osteoporosis;
         (c) Paget's disease;
         (d) osteoarthritis;
         (e) spinal stenosis.
(2) Enquire about previous back trouble, joint trouble, fever, weight loss, abdominal symptoms or urinary tract symptoms.
(3) Perform a full examination including an abdominal, rectal, neurological and breast examination and a urinalysis.
(4) X-ray the chest, thoracic and lumbosacral spine.

MANAGEMENT

Refer the patient to the appropriate specialist team according to the suspected aetiology.

NONTRAUMATIC — MILD TO MODERATE PAIN

DIAGNOSIS AND MANAGEMENT

(1) This rather nebulous group with no abnormal physical signs, apyrexial with a normal urinalysis may be allowed home.

(2) Prescribe a nonsteroidal anti-inflammatory analgesic such as diclofenac (Voltarol) 50 mg orally t.d.s.

(3) Give patients a letter for their general practitioner to follow them up and to arrange physiotherapy, an exercise regime and behaviour modification as appropriate.

REFERENCES

1   Stiell I.G., McKnight R.D., Greenberg G.H. *et al.* (1994). Implementation of the Ottawa ankle rules. *Journal of the American Medical Association*; **271**:827–832.

2   Senapati A. (1986). Conservative outpatient management of ingrowing toenails. *Journal of the Royal Society of Medicine*; **79**:339–340.

3   Malmivaara A., Häkkinen U., Aro T. *et al.* (1995). The treatment of acute low back pain — bed rest, exercises, or ordinary activity? *New England Journal of Medicine*; **332**:351–355.

PAEDIATRIC EMERGENCIES

Children account for a quarter to one-third of all patients seen in the A & E department. The total number of attendances is approximately double the number attending paediatric outpatients.

NORMAL VALUES

Until the doctor recognises the normal child, it is impossible to know what is abnormal and to identify sick patients.

(1) *Weight and height*:
   (i)   If the age is known, a simple formula for weight between age 1 and 10 years is:
         Weight (kg) = 2(Age + 4).
   (ii) Figure 11 enables an approximate weight to be derived from the age or length in centimetres (see page 265).
   (iii) Table 8 gives some normal values for weight and height.

(2) *Drug dosages*:
   (i)   Drugs should ideally be given on a per kilogram basis after weighing the child and consulting a drug formulary.
   (ii) Figure 11 is a paediatric resuscitation chart giving all commonly used emergency drugs in millilitres according to the age, weight or body length (see page 265).

(3) *Heart rate and blood pressure*:
   (i)   A formula for the normal blood pressure is:
         Systolic BP (mmHg) = 80 + 2(Age in years)
         Diastolic BP = 2/3 systolic BP.

Table 8. Normal values for weight and height

| Age (years) | Male | | Female | |
	Weight(kg)	Height(cm)	Weight(kg)	Height(cm)
Birth–1	3.5–10.3	50–75	3.4–9.6	50–74
2–5	12.5–19	85–107	12–18.5	84–106
5–12	19–38	107–147	18.5–40	106–149
14–16	49–60	160–172	51–56	160–162

Endotracheal tube

Oral length (cm)	Internal diameter (mm)
18–21	7.5–8.0 *cuffed*
18	7.0 *uncuffed*
17	6.5
16	6.0
15	5.5
14	5.0
13	4.5
12	4.0
	3.5
10	3.0–3.5

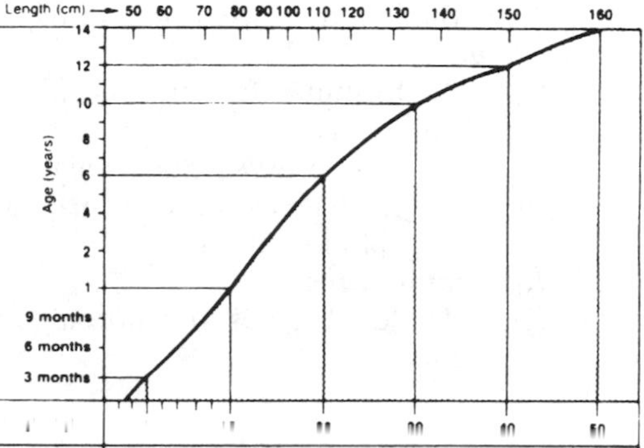

Adrenaline (ml of 1 in 10 000) *initial* *intravenous or intraosseous*	0.5	1	2	3	4	5
Adrenaline (ml of 1 in 1000) *subsequent* *intravenous or intraosseous (or initial endotracheal)*	0.5	1	2	3	4	5
• **Atropine (ml of 100 μg/ml)** *intravenous or intraosseous (or double if endotracheal)*	1	2	4	6	6	6
Atropine (ml) of 600 μg/ml)	–	0.3	0.7	1	1	1
Bicarbonate (ml of 8.4%) *intravenous or intraosseous (dilute to 4.2% in infants)*	5	10	20	30	40	50
• **Calcium chloride (ml of 10%)** *intravenous or intraosseous*	0.5	1	2	3	4	5
Diazepam (ml of 5 mg/ml *emulsion)* *intravenous or rectal*	0.4	0.8	1.6	2	2	2
Diazepam (mg *rectal tube solution)* *rectal*	*2.5 mg*	*5 mg*	*10 mg*	*10 mg*	*10 mg*	*10 mg*
Glucose (ml of 50%) *intravenous or intraosseous (dilute to 25% in infants)*	5	10	20	30	40	50
• **Lignocaine (ml of 1%)** *intravenous or intraosseous*	0.5	1	2	3	4	5
Naloxone *neonatal* (ml of 20 μg/ml) *intravenous or intraosseous*	2.5	5	–	–	–	–
Naloxone *adult* (ml of 400 μg/ml)	–	0.25	0.5	0.75	1	1.25
• **Salbutamol (mg** *nebulizer solution)* *via nebulizer (dilute to 2.5–5.0 ml in normal saline)*	–	*2.5 mg*	*5 mg*	*5 mg*	*5 mg*	*5 mg*
Initial DC defibrillation (J) *for VF or VT with no pulse*	*10*	*20*	*40*	*60*	*80*	*100*
Initial DC cardioversion (J) *for SVT with shock (synchronous)* *or VT with shock (non synchronous)*	*5*	*5*	*10*	*15*	*20*	*25*
Initial fluid bolus in shock (ml) *crystalloid or colloid*	100	200	400	600	800	1000

• ***CAUTION!*** *Non-standard drug concentrations may be available*
Use ***Atropine*** *100 μg/ml or prepare by diluting 1 mg to 10 ml or 600 μg to 6 ml in normal saline*
Note that 1 ml of ***calcium chloride*** *10% is equivalent to 3 ml of* ***calcium gluconate*** *10%*
Use ***Lignocaine*** *(without adrenaline) 1% or give twice the volume of 0.5%. Give half the volume of 2% or dilute appropriately*
Salbutamol may also be given by slow intravenous injection (5 μg/kg), but beware of the different concentrations available (eg 50 and 500 μg/ml)

Fig. 11. Paediatric Resuscitation Chart. Drug doses, endotracheal tube sizes and defibrillator settings are read off the chart according to the age, weight or body length, whichever is known. (Reproduced by kind permission of Peter Oakley, Anaesthesia/Trauma, Stoke-on-Trent.)

(ii)   Table 9 gives some normal values for the heart rate in the awake, active child and the blood pressure using a paediatric-sized cuff (two-thirds the length of the upper arm).

(4) *Circulatory blood volume*:

(i)   A formula for the normal circulatory blood volume is:

80–85 ml/kg body weight.

(ii)   Table 10 gives some normal values for the circulatory blood volume.

(5) *Respiratory rate*:

(i)   Table 11 gives the normal respiratory rate per minute.

Table 9. Normal values for heart rate and systolic blood pressure

Age (years)	Heart rate (beats per min)	Systolic BP (mmHg)
Under 1	110–160	70–90
2–5	95–140	80–100
5–12	80–120	90–110
Over 12	60–100	100–120

Table 10. Normal values for circulatory blood volume

Age (years)	Circulatory blood vol (ml)
Birth–1	300–800
2–5	990–1390
5–12	1390–2700
14–16	3500–4000

Table 11. Normal values for respiratory rate

Age (years)	Respiratory rate (per minute)
Under 1	30–40
2–5	20–30
5–12	15–20
Over 12	12–16

(6) *Developmental milestones*:
6 months:
  - (i)   sits erect with support;
  - (ii) localises sound 45 cm away;
  - (iii) alert and interested, friendly with strangers.

1 year:
  - (i)   crawls on all fours;
  - (ii) understands simple commands and babbles incessantly;
  - (iii) cooperates with dressing.

2 years:
  - (i)   runs and manages stairs;
  - (ii) joins words in simple phrases;
  - (iii) dry by day.

3 years:
  - (i)   can stand on one foot momentarily;
  - (ii) speaks in sentences;
  - (iii) dry by night.

5 years:
  - (i)   skips, hops and stands on one foot with ease;
  - (ii) fluent speech;
  - (iii) dresses and washes unaided.

11 years:
  appearance of pubic hair and breast buds in females.

12–13 years:
  appearance of pubic hair in males.

GENERAL CONSIDERATIONS

(1) The examination commences from the first moment the child is seen, whilst the parent or child is giving the history or the child alone is talking.

(2) Even infants and children unable to talk will give non-verbal cues about pain such as facial expression and posture.

(3) Most emergencies generate fear in children causing additional distress to the child and adding to parental anxiety.

(i)   Always explain things as clearly as possible, in such a way that the child can understand.

(ii)   Allow parents to stay with the child at all times.

(4) A complete examination of every child should include:

(i)   height, weight and head circumference measurements plotted on a percentile chart;

(ii)   an oral or rectal temperature (under 2 years);

(iii)   examination of the ear drums, mouth, throat (unless epiglottitis is suspected) and the skin;

(iv)   examination of a urine sample for sugar, protein and organisms, in all cases of abdominal pain, vomiting and drowsiness.

(5) Always refer the following potentially serious problems to the paediatric team, even if you are unable to reach a definite diagnosis yourself (see also under the management of a child with fever):

(i)   the quiet, pale child;

(ii)   the drowsy, or floppy child;

(iii)   the thin, malnourished child;

(iv)   the persistently crying child;

(v)   the child with difficulty in breathing;

(vi)   the child with stridor;

(vii)   the baby that has stopped feeding;

(viii)   the baby with repeated vomiting especially if it is bile-stained;

(ix)   the baby with frank blood mixed with the stools.

CARDIOPULMONARY RESUSCITATION

DIAGNOSIS

(1) Cardiac arrest in children is usually the end result of hypoxia, hypovolaemia and acidosis. Bradycardia progressing to asystole is almost invariable.

(2) The causes include:

(i)   Hypoxia from respiratory failure due to severe asthma, bronchiolitis, poisoning, near drowning or upper airway obstruction from epiglottitis, inhaled foreign body, etc;

    (ii)   Hypovolaemia due to haemorrhage, gastroenteritis, burns etc;

    (iii)   Septicaemia, anaphylaxis;

    (iv)   Sudden infant death syndrome.

(3) Ventricular fibrillation is uncommon but may occur in the following situations:

    (i)   Congenital heart disease;

    (ii)   Poisoning especially tricyclic antidepressant ingestion;

    (iii)   Hypothermia;

    (iv)   Myocarditis, cardiomyopathy and hereditary prolongation of the QT interval.

MANAGEMENT

Similar principles and practice apply as for adult resuscitation (see page 2). Refer to the Guidelines for Paediatric Life Support (see references).[1] Significant points of detail to note include:

(1) *Assisted ventilation.*

    (i)   In the event of a blocked airway from an inhaled foreign body, hold a small child prone and deliver five blows over the back, between the scapulae. An older child requires the Heimlich manoeuvre (see page 31).

    (ii)   Bag and mask ventilation is preferable to inexperienced attempts at intubation, which should be left to the anaesthetist.

        (a)   Insert an oropharyngeal (Guedel) airway measured from the centre of the mouth to the angle of the jaw when laid on the child's face. If it is too long it will damage the nasopharynx, and if too short it will push the tongue back. An airway is unnecessary in small babies.

        (b)   Position the head in a neutral position in infants under 1 year, as overextension of the head may actually occlude their airway.

        (c)   Use a face-mask that fits closely over the nose and mouth. Soft circular plastic masks are ideal.

(d) Attach a hand-ventilating device. The Laerdal Infant ventilating bag has a volume of 240 ml suitable for children up to 2 years, and is attached to an oxygen flow rate of at least 4 l/min. The Laerdal Child ventilating bag has a volume of 500 ml suitable for children up to 10 years.

(e) Inflate the chest at a faster rate than adults, up to 20 breaths per minute.

(iii) An endotracheal tube and both straight and curved blade laryngoscopes should be made ready for the anaesthetist or paediatrician and the tube cut to size (see Table 12).

(a) A rough guide to internal diameter tube size is:
Endotracheal tube size (mm) =
$$\frac{Age\ (yrs)}{4} + 4$$

(b) A rough guide to tube length is:
Oral endotracheal tube length (cm) =
$$\frac{Age\ (yrs)}{2} + 12$$
Nasal endotracheal tube length (cm) =
$$\frac{Age\ (yrs)}{2} + 15$$

Table 12. Correct size of orotracheal tube

Age	internal diameter (mm)	length (cm)
Birth	3.0	9
4 months	3.5	10
1 year	4.0	12
3 years	5.0	13
7 years	6.0	16
10 years	6.5	17
12 years	7.0 (+ cuff)	18
14 years	7.5 (+ cuff)	21
16 years	8.0 (+ cuff)	22
Adult	9.0 (+ cuff)	23

(2) *External cardiac massage.*

   (i)   In infants, use two fingers over the lower third of the sternum, depressing at a rate of at least 100/min.

   (ii)   In a child, use one hand at a rate of 100/min.

(3) *Venous access.*

   (i)   A 20-gauge or 22-gauge cannula is adequate, inserted into the most familiar site such as the antecubital fossa.

   (ii)   Connect this to an infusion of normal saline via a paediatric giving set slowed to a minimal rate, unless hypovolaemia is suspected when an initial fluid bolus of 20 ml/kg is rapidly given.

   (iii)   Other sites for venous access include the back of the hand, the external jugular, or the internal jugular vein if the doctor is suitably skilled.

   (iv)   If venous access is not gained within 90 s or 3 attempts, perform intraosseous (bone marrow) vascular access:

      (a) this may be used up to the age of 6 years;

      (b) use a specially designed intraosseous needle inserted into the anteromedial surface of the proximal tibia, 1–2 cm distal to the tuberosity;

      (c) advance the needle with a gentle twisting or boring motion until it gives on entering the marrow cavity and remove the stylet;

      (d) aspirate blood and marrow contents to confirm correct placement then connect an intravenous infusion giving set.

(4) *Drug administration.*

   (i)   If venous or intraosseous access is difficult, remember that adrenaline, atropine and lignocaine may be given via the endotracheal tube diluted in 2 ml normal saline:

      (a) adrenaline endotracheal dose is ten times the initial intravenous dose, i.e. 100 µg/kg:

      (b) atropine or lignocaine dose is twice the intravenous dose, i.e. 40 µg/kg and 2 mg/kg respectively.

(ii)   Recommended drug doses are:

Drug	Intravenous or intraosseous dosage
atropine (0.6 mg/ml)	20 µg or 0.03 ml/kg
adrenaline (1 in 10 000)	10 µg or 0.1 ml/kg
	100 µg or 1 ml/kg (second and subsequent doses)
bicarbonate (8.4%)	1 mmol or 1.0 ml/kg
calcium chloride (10%)	0.2 ml/kg
lignocaine 2% (100 mg/5 ml)	1 mg or 0.05 ml/kg
fluid (in hypovolaemia)	20 ml/kg

(iii)   Figure 11 is a paediatric resuscitation chart with all the drug doses calculated (see page 265).

(5) *Defibrillation.* Ventricular fibrillation is rare but has a better prognosis than asystole.
    (i)   Use paediatric paddles for children under 10 kg:
        (a)   These are 4.5 cm in diameter;
        (b)   If unavailable, use adult paddles placed on the infant's back and over the left lower front of chest.
    (ii)   Start at 2 J/kg for the first two shocks.
        (a)   Give 4 J/kg for third and subsequent shocks.

(6) *Heat loss.* Remember that in infants and small children considerable heat loss may occur, which will require overhead heating, an incubator, warming blankets and plastic sheets to cover exposed parts of the body.

(7) *When to stop.* The senior paediatric doctor will decide at which point further attempts are unlikely to be rewarding. He or she will also be responsible for the distressing duty of telling the parents.

COT DEATH (SUDDEN INFANT DEATH SYNDROME)

The cause of this syndrome is unknown although it is commoner in winter. The peak age is 3 months, with a higher incidence in bottle-fed males.

MANAGEMENT

(1) If the child is brought in by ambulance with resuscitation in progress, it is mandatory to continue this in the resuscitation room. Call the paediatric team urgently (see cardiopulmonary resuscitation, page 268).

(2) Examine the child carefully for any signs of trauma or infection, including evidence of asphyxia or of petechiae.

(3) Discuss the necessity for post-mortem blood tests for infection or a drug screen with the paediatric team. In addition, keep all clothes in a labelled hospital bag.

(4) The senior doctor should speak to the parents and encourage them to talk about the circumstances of the death and any recent illnesses.

    (i)   He or she should also explain the nature of the condition, the fact that it is unfortunately common, yet unexplained, and that no blame is attached to the parents, although it is normal for them to feel angry or guilty.

(5) Encourage the parents to see and hold their baby in privacy afterwards. They may derive benefit from the presence of the hospital chaplain and social worker.

(6) The parents must also be told that because the death is sudden the coroner's officer (or procurator fiscal in Scotland) will be informed, and a post mortem required.

(7) The coroner's officer or the police will then visit the parents later that day and will take further details, possibly even removing the bedding for examination.

(8) Write down and give the address and phone number of the Foundation for the Study of Infant Deaths to the parents so they can receive an information leaflet or arrange further counselling and support if they wish:

    Foundation for the Study of Infant Deaths
    35 Belgrave Square
    LONDON SW1X 8QB
    Telephone: 0171 235 1721 (24-h helpline).

(9) The doctor should also inform by telephone:

    (i)   the general practitioner to arrange for a home visit and to make certain all future clinic attendances for the deceased child are cancelled;

(ii)   the health visitor;
(iii)   the social work department;
(iv)   the paediatric team, if they were not present at the resuscitation;
(v)   the Community Child Health Department, to cancel immunisation appointments etc.

CHILD ABUSE (NONACCIDENTAL INJURY)

Various types are recognised, including physical and sexual abuse, poisoning and both social and emotional neglect.

DIAGNOSIS

(1) Maintain a high index of suspicion in the following circumstances, especially in children under 4 years old:
   (i)   History:
          (a)   a delay between the alleged injury and the presentation to the A & E department;
          (b)   inconsistency between the story and the actual injuries;
          (c)   abnormal parental behaviour, poor interaction with the child and apparent lack of parental concern;
          (d)   frequent attendance in the A & E department (by the child or a sibling), often for little apparent reason;
          (e)   previous injuries on different dates;
          (f)   failure to thrive, or signs of neglect.
   (ii)   Examination:
          The child must be fully undressed in stages to be examined completely and all findings are carefully documented. Measure bruises, scratches, burns and other skin marks with a ruler. Polaroid photos provide useful contemporaneous evidence. Look specifically for:

(a) Torn upper-lip frenulum, or palatal haemorrhage from a feeding bottle or even a fist thrust into the mouth to prevent the baby crying, or from a direct blow.

(b) Human bite marks, and bruising from a fist or slapping, which may rupture the tympanic membrane.

(c) Deep cigarette burns, or scalds limited to the buttocks and genitalia or both feet, suggesting immersion in hot water.

(d) A fractured skull or long bone particularly in a child not yet able to walk. A spiral fracture of a long bone is most suspicious, as are other healing fractures of differing ages on skeletal survey.

(e) Subconjunctival, vitreous or retinal haemorrhage suggesting violent shaking, or from a direct blow.

(f) Signs of sexual abuse to the genitalia or anus.

MANAGEMENT

(1) If you have any suspicion of child abuse inform the paediatric team immediately and arrange for admission of the child. Check if the child is on the child abuse register already.

(2) Do not confront the parent at this stage, but explain that you want a further opinion from a senior paediatric doctor.

(3) If the parent refuses admission, contact the social work department. If necessary they can apply to a magistrate for an 8-day emergency protection order, with the right of challenge for parents after 72 h

(4) In an emergency, the police can act without requiring a magistrate's order to take a child into protection for up to 72 h.

Note: remember that osteogenesis imperfecta presents as multiple fractures, and idiopathic thrombocytopenic purpura and leukaemia cause multiple bruising and bleeding. However, these are rare compared with the genuine cases of child abuse.

THE BREATHLESS CHILD

The causes and management of stridor are dealt with in the next chapter. Important causes of a breathless child are:
 (1) bronchiolitis;
 (2) bronchitis;
 (3) pneumonia;
 (4) asthma;
 (5) inhaled foreign body;
 (6) allergic and metabolic conditions.

BRONCHIOLITIS

DIAGNOSIS

 (1) This condition occurs in seasonal epidemics, affecting babies under 1 year old, commonly due to the respiratory syncytial virus.
 (2) It starts with fever and snuffles, but rapidly progresses to cough, irritability, fluid refusal, wheeze and marked tachypnoea.
 (3) Expiratory rhonchi and fine crepitations are heard in the chest which may appear hyperinflated, and in extreme cases cyanosis develops with a raised respiratory rate and intercostal recession.

MANAGEMENT

 (1) Give the child oxygen, attach a pulse oximeter and admit under the paediatric team particularly if there has been poor feeding, respiratory recession, apnoea or cyanosis.
 (2) Request a portable CXR or x-ray on the way to the ward, with a nurse or doctor in attendance. Hyperinflation with small areas of atelectasis may be the only abnormalities seen.

BRONCHITIS

DIAGNOSIS AND MANAGEMENT

(1) This causes fever, cough and wheeze.
(2) It may be the early feature of measles.
(3) Refer the child to the paediatric team following a CXR.

PNEUMONIA

DIAGNOSIS AND MANAGEMENT

(1) *Bronchopneumonia* occurs in young children, or older children with chronic illness, e.g. cerebral palsy, and may be bacterial or viral. There is cough, fever and dyspnoea.
(2) *Lobar pneumonia* presents with sudden illness, fever, breathlessness and pleuritic chest pain.
(3) *Staphylococcal pneumonia* occurs in infants and in older children with cystic fibrosis and presents with septicaemia, pneumothorax, empyema, etc.
(4) Remember that the nonspecific presenting features of pneumonia include fever, lethargy, anorexia, abdominal pain or meningism.
(5) X-ray all the above cases and refer to the paediatric team for oxygen, fluids, antibiotics and nursing care.

ASTHMA

DIAGNOSIS

(1) Reversible airways obstruction in children is associated with infection (usually viral), allergy, atopy, exercise and emotion.
(2) It is one of the commonest reasons for admission to hospital in childhood.
(3) Asthma presents with wheezing, prolonged expiratory dyspnoea and cough. A similar assessment as for adults is made, including a pulse, respiratory rate and peak flow before treatment (see page 26).
(4) A severe attack is indicated by any of the following:

    (i)   too breathless to talk;
    (ii)   too breathless to feed;
    (iii)   respiratory rate 50 or more breaths per minute;
    (iv)   tachycardia 140 or more beats per minute;
    (v)   peak expiratory flow rate 50% or less of predicted or best.

MANAGEMENT

(1) Sit the child up and give oxygen, ideally with the mother in attendance to reassure the child. Attach a pulse oximeter, aiming for an oxygen saturation above 92%.

(2) Give nebulised salbutamol 2.5–5 mg diluted to 5 ml with saline, using an oxygen-driven delivery system.

(3) Add ipratropium (Atrovent) 125–250 µg to the next nebuliser if the salbutamol is ineffective, then continue the nebulised salbutamol up to half-hourly until improved.

(4) Refer all cases to the paediatric team, and discuss with them the indications for a CXR, and oral prednisolone 1 mg/kg which shortens the duration of the acute attack.

INHALED FOREIGN BODY

DIAGNOSIS AND MANAGEMENT

(1) This may present as upper airway obstruction with stridor or with sudden coughing and wheeze.

(2) If the object passes into the lower airways, all symptoms may disappear. Later wheeze, infection or obstructive emphysema supervene, causing localised rhonchi, crepitations and breathlessness.

(3) Request a PA and lateral CXR. Although organic foreign bodies such as peanuts will not show, the secondary effects of compensatory hyperinflation on an expiratory film, collapse and consolidation will gradually appear.

(4) Refer the child to the paediatric team.

ALLERGIC AND METABOLIC CONDITIONS

DIAGNOSIS AND MANAGEMENT

(1) Drug allergy to salicylates, antibiotics, etc. may present as breathlessness and wheeze as part of angioneurotic oedema or an anaphylactic reaction. Management is similar to that for adults (see page 106).

(2) Diabetic ketoacidosis presents with deep, sighing respirations; peritonitis with rapid, shallow breathing. The child will be severely ill and other features will alert the doctor to the underlying diagnosis.

(3) Refer all these patients immediately to the paediatric team.

STRIDOR

This is noise predominantly on inspiration originating from airway obstruction above the level of the larynx. There are three important causes:

(1) acute laryngotracheobronchitis or 'croup';
(2) epiglottitis;
(3) inhaled foreign body.

ACUTE LARYNGOTRACHEOBRONCHITIS (CROUP)

DIAGNOSIS AND MANAGEMENT

(1) Croup usually occurs between the ages of 1 and 3 years due to a virus such as parainfluenza.

(2) Hoarseness, a barking cough and harsh inspiratory stridor develop, typically in the middle of the night, preceded by an upper respiratory tract infection.

(3) The child is irritable and tired but lacks the drooling, dysphagia and toxic appearance of epiglottitis.

(4) Refer all cases to the paediatric team for admission for observation, humidified oxygen, and nebulised or systemic steroids.

(5) Nebulised 1 in 1000 adrenaline 5 ml produces transient improvement in the most severe cases, who must all be admitted to ITU.[2]

EPIGLOTTITIS

DIAGNOSIS

(1) This is a life-threatening illness with sudden onset of sore throat, dysphagia and difficulty in breathing usually due to *Haemophilus influenzae.*
(2) The child looks severely ill, pale and sits up leaning forwards, drooling. The voice is muffled and the stridor softer than with croup.

MANAGEMENT

(1) Do not examine the child further. Do not request or perform a rectal temperature, BP or x-ray and do not attempt to visualise the throat.
(2) Leave the child with the parent, sitting upright with an oxygen mask held near its face.
(3) Summon urgent senior paediatric, anaesthetic and ENT help, and warn ITU.
(4) Stay with the child until help arrives. If sudden respiratory arrest occurs, be prepared to attempt intubation with a small endotracheal tube and an introducer. If this fails, insert a large-bore intravenous cannula through the cricothyroid membrane as an emergency airway (see page 31).

INHALED FOREIGN BODY

DIAGNOSIS

(1) There is sudden onset of cough, spluttering and choking noises, appropriate to the degree of airway obstruction. Hoarseness or aphonia may occur.

(2) The child may progress to complete airway obstruction, remain unchanged or all the symptoms may disappear as the foreign body passes into the lower airways.

MANAGEMENT

(1) Complete airway obstruction:
   (i)   Hold small children head down and deliver blows to the back between the shoulder blades.
   (ii) In older children perform the Heimlich manoeuvre (see page 31).
   (iii) If the above two fail, attempt removal of the impacted object using a laryngoscope and a pair of long-handled forceps, or proceed directly to emergency cricothyrotomy (see page 31).

(2) Stable airway obstruction:
   (i)   Summon urgent anaesthetic and ENT help.
   (ii) Await their arrival before considering a lateral soft-tissue x-ray of the neck or a CXR.

(3) Disappearance of the symptoms of obstruction:
   (i)   Consider the possibility that the foreign body has passed further into the lower airways.
   (ii) Request a PA and lateral CXR if the object is radio-opaque.
   (iii) Otherwise, if the object is radiolucent, request an inspiratory and expiratory CXR. Look for compensatory hyperinflation on the expiratory film, or the development of collapse and consolidation.
   (iv) Refer the child to the paediatric team if the history is convincing, even when the CXR appears normal.

ABDOMINAL PAIN, DIARRHOEA AND VOMITING

Abdominal pain may present acutely, or become chronic and recurrent. Diarrhoea and vomiting are common problems which may both lead to dehydration.

ACUTE ABDOMINAL PAIN

DIAGNOSIS

(1) *History.*

    (i)   Ask about the onset of the pain, the site, duration and previous similar episodes.

    (ii)   Enquire about associated vomiting or diarrhoea, and the time of the last bowel motion or the passage of flatus.

    (iii)   Record any medication given or known allergy.

    (iv)   Children aged over 2 years should be able to indicate the site of their pain. In infants, pain may be inferred from spasms of crying, restlessness, drawing up of the knees and refusal to feed.

(2) *Examination.*

    (i)   The whole child should be examined fully undressed to search for signs of a raised temperature, rash, upper respiratory tract infection, and localising signs in the abdomen including inspection of the genitalia.

    (ii)   The urine must always be examined for sugar and, if pyelonephritis is suspected, it should be sent for microscopy and culture.

        (a)   White cells may also be seen in the urine in pelvic peritonitis and appendicitis.

    (iii)   Erect and supine abdominal films are requested for suspected intestinal obstruction.

(3) *Causes of acute abdominal pain.*

These are best considered in two groups.

    (i)   Surgical:

        (a) appendicitis;

        (b) Meckel's diverticulitis;

        (c) peritonitis;

        (d) intestinal obstruction including intussusception and sigmoid volvulus;

        (e) strangulated inguinal hernia;

        (f) testicular torsion.

    (ii)   *Medical*:

        (a) mesenteric adenitis;

        (b) gastroenteritis;

(c) urinary tract infection;
(d) hepatitis;
(e) diabetic ketoacidosis;
(f) pneumonia;
(g) tonsillitis;
(h) meningitis;
(i) Henoch–Schönlein purpura.

MANAGEMENT

(1) Ideally refer all cases to the paediatric team.
(2) Significant features include pain for over 3 h, associated pyrexia and vomiting.
(3) If the child is allowed home, inform the general practitioner by telephone and letter and arrange for review of the child the next morning.

RECURRENT ABDOMINAL PAIN

DIAGNOSIS

(1) The vast majority of cases (over 90%) do not appear to have an organic cause, but remember the possibility of:
   (i) urinary tract infection and hydronephrosis;
   (ii) inflammatory bowel disease;
   (iii) recurrent volvulus;
   (iv) peptic ulcer.
(2) Recurrent abdominal pain of childhood or 'periodic syndrome' is the usual cause. A child with this condition may, however, present with a new acute organic illness at any time.

MANAGEMENT

(1) Examine the child fully as for an acute attack of abdominal pain.
(2) Refer the child back to the general practitioner if nothing is found, or to the paediatric outpatient department.
(3) Instruct the parents to return with the child at the start of the next attack of abdominal pain.

DIARRHOEA, VOMITING AND DEHYDRATION

DIAGNOSIS

(1) Diarrhoea and vomiting are common problems that require investigation and treatment. Dehydration is a serious end result.

(2) *Causes of diarrhoea.*

    (i)   Gastroenteritis: this is usually viral due to a rotavirus, but it can be due to *Escherichia coli*, or *Salmonella*, etc.

    (ii)   Surgical conditions such as appendicitis, peritonitis or occasionally intussusception.

    (iii)   Drugs, e.g. ampicillin.

    (iv)   Other infections such as tonsillitis or otitis media.

    (v)   Malabsorption, ulcerative colitis, Crohn's disease.

    (vi)   Dietary indiscretion, including too much or too little food.

    (vii) 'Toddler diarrhoea'.

(3) *Causes of vomiting.*

    (i)   Causes in the newborn:

        (a) infection, including meningitis and UTI;

        (b) intestinal obstruction from duodenal atresia, Hirschsprung's disease or a meconium plug;

        (c) cerebral haemorrhage or oedema;

        (d) metabolic, such as galactosaemia or congenital adrenal hyperplasia.

    (ii)   Causes in infants (up to 1 year):

        (a) pyloric stenosis, typically in males aged 3–8 weeks;

        (b) infections including gastroenteritis, tonsillitis, otitis media, meningitis and UTI;

        (c) intestinal obstruction from intussusception, or an obstructed hernia, etc.;

        (d) gastro-oesophageal reflux and hiatus hernia;

        (e) feeding problems due to overfeeding or excessive wind;

        (f) poisoning.

    (iii)   Causes after infancy:

        (a) infections – see (ii) (b) above;

        (b) intestinal obstruction or appendicitis;

    (c) metabolic, such as ketoacidosis or uraemia;
    (d) raised intracranial pressure;
    (e) migraine or periodic syndrome;
    (f) poisoning.

MANAGEMENT

(1) Take a careful history and examine for the above possible causes. Refer any patient with suggestive features to the paediatric team for investigation.

(2) *Assessment of dehydration.*
Regardless of the suspected cause, dehydration requires assessment and treating in its own right:

    (i)   Mild dehydration (less than 5% body weight lost): the child is in good general condition with dry mouth, thirst and mild oliguria.

    (ii)   Moderate dehydration (5–10%): the child looks ill, is floppy and apathetic with sunken eyes and fontanelle, has a dry mouth, decreased skin tissue turgor, tachycardia, marked thirst and oliguria.

    (iii) Severe dehydration (10% or more body weight lost): the child is drowsy, cool, cyanosed, tachypnoeic, tachycardic, hypotense and may become comatose. There is a risk of sudden death.

Note: beware missing the diagnosis of dehydration in an overweight baby presenting with tachycardia alone.

(3) *Treatment of mild dehydration.*
    (i)   Stop all milk and solid food for 24 h (breastfeeding is continued supplemented by extra water or glucose-electrolyte solution between feeds).

    (ii)   Use an oral glucose-electrolyte solution, e.g. Dioralyte or Rehidrat:

        (a) make up the sachet with water according to the instructions and in infants give 1–1½ times the volume of their usual feed;

        (b) in older children, give 200 ml of solution after each loose motion, or enough to quench the thirst, given in frequent small amounts;

(c) aim to replace the normal maintenance fluid requirement, plus an extra 20–50% fluid to cover continuing losses;

(d) normal maintenance fluid requirement per hour according to the usual body weight is:

Up to 10 kg	4 ml/kg
10–20 kg	40 ml + (2 ml/kg for each kg over 10 kg)
Over 20 kg	60 ml + (1 ml/kg for each kg over 20 kg)

(iii) After 24–48 h, begin graduated feeds with half-strength milk for a day in infants, and a bland diet gradually reintroducing solids in the older child.

(iv) Give the parents a letter for the general practitioner and instruct them to return if the child's condition deteriorates.

(4) *Treatment of moderate or severe dehydration.*

(i) Send blood for U&E, blood sugar and FBC and start an infusion of half-normal (0.45%) saline giving 20–25 ml/kg over 1–2 h, whilst waiting for the electrolyte results.

(a) If the child is shocked, give 20 ml/kg of a plasma expander such as polygeline (Haemaccel) rapidly over 10–20 mins, repeated as necessary to restore the circulation.

(ii) Further fluid management will depend on the blood results and degree of dehydration. If the child has hypernatraemic dehydration, fluid and electrolyte replacement must be given slowly over 2–3 days to avoid seizures due to cerebral oedema.

(iii) Refer the child to the paediatric team for immediate admission.

FEVER

The normal oral temperature is 37°C, and the normal rectal temperature is 37.5°C. A fever is defined as a rectal temperature above 38°C.

Table 13. Common childhood exanthematous diseases

Disease	Incubation period (days)	Prodrome	Rash	Other features and infectivity
Chickenpox	10–20	None	Macules, papules, vesicles and pustules of differing ages	Infective until all vesicles are crusted over (usually 6 days after last crop)
Glandular fever	5–14	Fever, sore throat, malaise	Transient maculopapular (rare); itchy drug rash with ampicillin (common)	Palatal petechiae, cervical lymphadenopathy; hepatosplenomegaly; tonsillar exudate; infective for many months by close physical contact
Measles	9–14	3 days of cough, cold and conjunctivitis	Red, confluent, maculopapular, lasts 7–11 days	Koplik's spots; cough predominates; may be quite ill; infective for 5 days after rash appears
Rubella	14–21	None	Pink, maculopapular discrete; lasts 3–5 days	Occipital and preauricular lymphadenopathy; infective until rash disappears
Scarlet fever	2–5	1–2 days sore throat, fever, vomiting	Minute, red, punctate papules; lasts 7 days	Unwell; circumoral pallor; 'strawberry tongue'; infective until negative throat swabs following penicillin

DIAGNOSIS

(1) Look for the following common causes of fever in a child:
   (i)   upper and lower respiratory tract infection;
   (ii)   otitis media;
   (iii)   tonsillitis;
   (iv)   viral exanthema, even before the rash appears (see Table 13);
   (v)   UTI;
   (vi)   appendicitis;
   (vii)   meningitis and septicaemia;
   (viii) malaria, particularly if the child has been abroad to an endemic area in the previous 2 years.
(2) Serious bacterial infections including meningitis, septicaemia, bone and joint infections, UTI, pneumonia and enteritis may all present with fever and no localising signs.[3]

MANAGEMENT

(1) Refer the following febrile patients to the paediatric team, even if you are unable to find a definite source:
   (i)   children aged under 6 months, particularly if they are drowsy, pale, have difficulty in breathing or have taken less than half their normal feeds over 24 h or produced less than 4 wet nappies in 24 h.
   (ii)   children under 3 years who appear toxic, e.g. are lethargic, poorly perfused and hypoventilating or hyperventilating.
   (iii)   children with a temperature of 40°C or more;
   (iv)   any signs of meningism, irritability, drowsiness or a history of seizure (see page 49);
   (v)   an unexplained rash particularly if petechial or purpuric;
   (vi)   any signs of dehydration (see page 285).
(2) If there is no obvious cause for a fever, send a specimen of urine for culture and, if the child is not ill and does not fulfil any of the above criteria, advise the parents to adopt symptomatic measures including:

    (i)   regular fluid intake — 'little but often';

    (ii)   minimal clothing;

    (iii)   paracetamol elixir at a dose of 15 mg/kg 4-hourly (paracetamol oral suspension is available in two strengths with either 120 mg paracetamol/5 ml or 250 mg paracetamol/5 ml).

(3) Always write a letter to the general practitioner indicating your findings, even if they were negative, and arrange for the child to be seen again within 24 h.

FITS AND FEBRILE CONVULSIONS

FITS

Fits must be distinguished from other causes of brief loss of consciousness such as syncope, pallid breath-holding and cyanotic breath-holding.

DIAGNOSIS

Consider the likely cause of the fit according to the age of the child:

(1) *Newborn*. Seizures tend to be mere twitching of a limb, fluttering of an eyelid or conjugate eye deviation. Causes include:

    (i)   hypoglycaemia;

    (ii)   hypocalcaemia;

    (iii)   hypoxia, especially from birth injury;

    (iv)   cerebral haemorrhage and subdural haematoma;

    (v)   infection.

(2) *Preschool child*.

    (i)   The commonest cause is a febrile convulsion. Other possibilities include:

    (ii)   idiopathic epilepsy;

    (iii)   sudden reduction in epilepsy medication;

    (iv)   meningitis or encephalitis;

    (v)   head injury (including injury from child abuse);

    (vi)   dehydration from gastroenteritis, etc.;

(vii) hypoglycaemia;
(viii) poisoning.
(3) *Older child*. Causes include:
    (i)   idiopathic epilepsy;
    (ii)   sudden reduction in epilepsy medication;
    (iii) head injury;
    (iv) hypoglycaemia;
    (v)   poisoning, including lead, iron and tricyclic antidepressants.

MANAGEMENT

(1) Clear the airway, place the child on its side and give oxygen via a face mask.
(2) Check for hypoglycaemia using a Glucostix and if the reading is low, give 2 ml/kg of 25% dextrose i.v. having saved 1 ml serum for subsequent laboratory blood glucose estimation.
(3) Record the rectal temperature and if it is raised, tepid sponge the child and use a fan.
(4) If the child fits again or is still fitting:
    (i)   Give rectal diazepam 0.5 mg/kg with full resuscitation equipment available should respiratory depression or hypotension occur.
        (a) Use either the parenteral diazepam solution (Valium) given via a syringe with a short, plastic catheter or
        (b) use the proprietary rectal tube (Stesolid) available as 5 mg or 10 mg diazepam per 2.5 ml tube.
    (ii)   Gain intravenous access and if the child is still fitting, give intravenous diazepam (Diazemuls) 0.1–0.2 mg/kg at 1 mg/min up to a maximum of 0.5 mg/kg.
    (iii) If intravenous access is impossible, an alternative is paraldehyde:
        (a) give 0.3 ml/kg rectally diluted 1:10 with normal saline or vegetable oil;
        (b) or give 0.15 ml/kg deep intramuscularly into two different sites, if the volume is over 2 ml.

There is a risk of a subsequent painful, local sterile abscess (check current prescribing information with manufacturer).

(5) Refer all children with a fit to the paediatric team. Intravenous phenytoin 18 mg/kg will be required for recurrent or persistent fits.

FEBRILE CONVULSIONS

These are the commonest cause of fits in preschool children.

DIAGNOSIS

(1) Features that favour the diagnosis of febrile convulsion are:
   (i)   age between 6 months and 5 years;
   (ii) the child is unwell before the fit with a rising temperature;
   (iii) a generalised, nonfocal fit that lasts under 10 minutes;
   (iv) a fit that does not recur (except a few hours after the first), and that does not leave any focal neurological signs, or residual weakness such as a Todd's palsy.

(2) If there are features different from the above, the episode should not be labelled a febrile convulsion.

MANAGEMENT

(1) Undress the child, tepid-sponge and use a fan.
(2) Insert paracetamol 15 mg/kg as a suppository.
(3) Refer the child to the paediatric team.

ACUTE POISONING

Most cases of acute poisoning in children are accidental, although rarely deliberate poisoning may occur as a form of child abuse and adolescents may attempt suicide.

DIAGNOSIS

(1) Three categories of substances may be taken:
   (i)   proprietary tablets and syrups, often prescribed for the parents;
   (ii)   household and garden chemicals;
   (iii) leaves, berries, seeds and fungi.
(2) It is important to ascertain what was taken, how much and when. If possible, the container the poison was in should be brought with the child, or an example of the flora ingested.
(3) Baseline observations of temperature, pulse, blood pressure, respiratory rate, level of consciousness and a Glucostix for hypoglycaemia, particularly in alcohol and salicylate poisoning, are recorded.

MANAGEMENT

(1) Institute urgent treatment to save life, including clearing the airway and giving oxygen. If the gag reflex is absent, use a bag and mask with an oropharyngeal airway and call the anaesthetist urgently to intubate the child.
(2) If the Glucostix reads low, give 2 ml/kg of 25% dextrose i.v.
(3) If there are pinpoint pupils and respiratory depression, give naloxone 10 μg/kg i.v. (or via the endotracheal tube or i.m. if venous access is impossible), followed by naloxone 100 μg/kg i.v. if no response.
(4) Start an intravenous infusion of normal saline for hypotension, and send blood for U&E, blood sugar and a drug screen which may include a salicylate, paracetamol, iron, theophylline or alcohol level.
(5) Otherwise, if the child is conscious, induce emesis if serious poisoning is suspected:
   (i)   Give syrup of ipecacuanha 10 ml up to 18 months of age, or 15 ml if the child is older, followed by 100–200 ml of water or orange juice. Repeat this in 20 min if there is no response.
   (ii)   Contraindications to ipecacuanha are:
       (a) ingestion of corrosive material, paraffin or petrol;
       (b) altered level of consciousness.

(iii) The use of ipecacuanha is declining, but may be acceptable if given early by a parent at home prior to arrival in hospital.

(6) Gastric lavage is rarely indicated or performed, except in potentially lethal poisoning presenting early.
  (i) Call the anaesthetist to protect the airway first by endotracheal intubation.
  (ii) The same contraindications concerning corrosives, paraffin and petrol apply to gastric lavage.

(7) Activated charcoal 1 g/kg is being increasingly used to reduce the absorption of many poisons. It is unpalatable and difficult to administer in children, but may be given via a nasogastric tube (see page 66).

(8) Refer all patients to the paediatric team, even if there are no initial symptoms nor signs

(9) Advice and help is available from the various Poisons Information Centres (see page 67), and from local botanical departments for plant identification.

(10) Specific poisonings and their treatment are described on pages 67–79, in the chapter on acute poisoning in adults.

THE LIMPING CHILD

DIFFERENTIAL DIAGNOSIS

(1) Exclude trivial local causes like a painful shoe, verruca, foreign body in the foot or groin lymphadenopathy.

(2) Hip pain is referred to the knee and vice versa, so always examine both.

(3) Typical causes according to age are listed below:
  (i) Age 0–5 years:
    (a) congenital dislocation of the hip;
    (b) transient synovitis 'irritable hip'.
  (ii) 5–10 years: Perthes' disease.
  (iii) 10–15 years: slipped upper femoral epiphysis.
  (iv) Any age:
    (a) trauma;

    (b) osteomyelitis, septic arthritis (including TB);
    (c) Still's disease and leukaemia.

MANAGEMENT

(1) X-ray all these children and refer to the orthopaedic team, if the limp is confirmed and an innocent local cause is not found.
(2) Ultrasound is useful to demonstrate a hip effusion and if positive, may be followed by aspiration under anaesthesia to exclude a septic arthritis.

REFERENCES

1   Paediatric Life Support Working Party of the European Resuscitation Council (1994). Guidelines for Paediatric Life Support. *British Medical Journal*; **308**:1349–1355.
2   Advanced Life Support Group (1993). *Advanced Paediatric Life Support*, 1st edn. London: BMJ Publishing Group.
3   Baraff L.J., Bass J.W., Fleisher G.R. *et al.* (1993). Practice guideline for the management of infants and children 0–36 months of age with fever without source. *Annals of Emergency Medicine*; **22**:1198–1210.

ENT EMERGENCIES

TRAUMATIC CONDITIONS OF THE EAR

SUBPERICHONDRIAL HAEMATOMA

DIAGNOSIS

(1) Blunt trauma to the ear causes bleeding between the auricular cartilage and perichondrium, known as a subperichondrial haematoma.
(2) If untreated this will lead to a 'cauliflower ear' deformity from proliferative fibrosis.

MANAGEMENT

(1) Aspirate small clots under local anaesthesia and apply firm pressure by packing around the interstices of the ear with cotton-wool under a turban dressing. Refer the patient to the next ENT clinic, since the bleeding may recur.
(2) Protect against perichondritis with flucloxacillin 500 mg orally q.d.s. for 5 days.
(3) Refer the patient with a large and extensive bleed directly to the ENT team for immediate drainage through multiple small incisions.

WOUNDS OF THE AURICLE

MANAGEMENT

(1) Perform minimal debridement of devitalised tissue under local anaesthesia.
(2) Refer the patient to the ENT team or plastic surgeons, if there is skin loss leaving exposed cartilage or extensive lacerations.
(3) Otherwise, appose the edges of the cartilage with 5/0 chromic catgut or polyglactin (Vicryl) through the perichondrium.
(4) Then suture the skin with 6/0 synthetic monofilament and apply a firm dressing. Remove the sutures after 7 days.

(5) Protect against perichondritis with flucloxacillin 500 mg orally q.d.s. for 5 days and give tetanus prophylaxis.

FOREIGN BODY IN THE EXTERNAL EAR

DIAGNOSIS AND MANAGEMENT

(1) A foreign body in the external ear causes pain, deafness and discharge if left.
(2) If the foreign body is superficial, attempt gentle removal with a loop or blunt right-angle probe.
(3) (i)   Do not attempt any further manoeuvres if the object is not freed instantly, or if the patient is uncooperative, as the object may be pushed further in and the eardrum damaged.
    (ii)   Refer the patient to the next ENT clinic.

PERFORATED EARDRUM

DIAGNOSIS

(1) The eardrum may be perforated by direct injury from a sharp object like a hairpin, or indirectly by pressure from a slap, blast injury, from SCUBA diving, or from a fracture of the base of the skull (see below).
(2) There is pain, conductive deafness and sometimes bleeding.
(3) If there is severe vertigo or complete hearing loss, suspect inner ear involvement.

MANAGEMENT

(1) Refer the patient immediately to the ENT team if inner ear damage is suspected.
(2) Otherwise, do not put anything into the ear or attempt to clean it out. Advise the patient to keep water out of the ear canal.
(3) Give an antibiotic such as amoxycillin 500 mg orally t.d.s. and refer the patient to the next ENT clinic.

BASAL SKULL FRACTURE

Most basal skull fractures (see also page 130) involve the temporal bone. Its fractures may be divided into tympanic bone fracture, longitudinal and transverse fractures.

DIAGNOSIS

(1) The temporal bone forms the glenoid fossa of the temporomandibular joint, and is damaged if the mandibular condyle is driven upwards into the middle ear or external auditory canal, causing bleeding or laceration of the canal.

(2) Alternatively, a longitudinal fracture of the temporal bone will tear the eardrum and cause dislocation of the ossicular chain, with conductive deafness, haemotympanum and CSF leakage. Occasionally delayed facial nerve damage is seen.

(3) A transverse fracture of the temporal bone results in complete sensorineural deafness associated with tinnitus, nystagmus and vertigo. Facial nerve palsy is more common than with longitudinal fractures.

MANAGEMENT

(1) Do not insert an auriscope to examine obvious bleeding from the external auditory meatus, as infection may be introduced.

(2) Remember that basal skull fracture is a clinical diagnosis. X-rays may have to wait until the patient is stabilised on the ward and other injuries to the head, neck and chest have been fully assessed.

    (i) Intracranial air or a fluid level in the sphenoid sinus on lateral skull x-ray are suggestive of a fracture.

    (ii) Request an immediate CT scan providing the patient has been stabilised.

(3) Admit the patient under the surgical team for head injury care and subsequent advice from the ENT specialist or neurosurgical unit.

NONTRAUMATIC CONDITIONS OF THE EAR

All these conditions present with pain and/or hearing loss.

OTITIS EXTERNA

DIAGNOSIS

(1) A bacterial or fungal infection, often following exposure to water, is usually responsible ('swimmer's ear').
(2) There is pain, desquamation of skin, and a thin, offensive discharge that may become frankly purulent.

MANAGEMENT

(1) Perform aural toilet using a cotton wick to gently remove the debris.
(2) Give the patient a proprietary anti-infective and steroid preparation, e.g. 1% clioquinol with 0.02% flumethasone (Locorten-Vioform) 3 drops b.d. to the external auditory canal.
(3) Refer the patient to the ENT clinic for follow-up.
(4) If the otitis externa is severe, with occlusion of the canal, refer the patient directly to the ENT team.

FURUNCULOSIS OF THE EXTERNAL EAR

DIAGNOSIS

(1) A furuncle may develop in the outer part of the external auditory canal causing extreme pain.
(2) Movement of the pinna and introduction of a speculum exacerbate the pain. Deafness is minimal.

MANAGEMENT

(1) Insert a wick soaked in 10% ichthammol in glycerine to encourage discharge of the pus, start flucloxacillin 500 mg

orally q.d.s. and an analgesic such as paracetamol 500 mg and codeine phosphate 8 mg (co-codamol) two tablets orally q.d.s. Refer the patient to the ENT clinic for follow-up.

(2) Test the urine for sugar.

ACUTE OTITIS MEDIA

DIAGNOSIS

(1) This is common in children due to pneumococcus or *Haemophilus influenzae* (in children under 6 years).

(2) There is intense earache, conductive deafness, fever and, on examining the eardrum in the early stages, there is loss of the light reflex and injected vessels are seen around the malleus.

(3) As the infection progresses, a bulging drum is seen, that may perforate, discharging pus.

MANAGEMENT

(1) In the early stages give amoxycillin 250–500 mg orally t.d.s. for 5 days and an analgesic such as paracetamol elixir 15 mg/kg 4-hourly.

(2) Use erythromycin 250–500 mg orally q.d.s. for 5 days if the patient is allergic to penicillin.

(3) If the drum is bulging or has perforated and the child is unwell, refer directly to the ENT team.

MASTOIDITIS

DIAGNOSIS AND MANAGEMENT

(1) There is extension of infection from acute otitis media into the mastoid air-cell system.

(2) The patient is ill and feverish, with tenderness over the mastoid and the pinna is pushed down and forwards.

(3) Refer the patient immediately to the ENT team for x-ray, CT scan and parenteral antibiotics.

(4) Complications include cranial nerve palsy, meningitis and subperiosteal abscess.

VERTIGO

DIAGNOSIS

(1) Two main groups occur.
- (i) *Central vertigo*: This is due to lesions in the CNS, such as a vertebrobasilar TIA, cerebellar or brain-stem stroke, cerebral tumour, demyelination, vertebrobasilar migraine and drug toxicity.
- (ii) *Peripheral vertigo*: This is due to lesions in the vestibular nerve and inner ear, such as vestibular neuronitis, Ménière's disease, benign paroxysmal positional vertigo, acoustic neuroma, otosclerosis, cholesteatoma and ototoxic drugs.

(2) Central vertigo is usually dominated by associated neurological signs, whereas peripheral vertigo causes nystagmus, deafness, nausea, vomiting and sweating.

MANAGEMENT

(1) Incapacitating vertigo may be controlled by diazepam (Diazemuls) 5–10 mg i.v. or prochlorperazine (Stemetil) 12.5 mg i.m.
(2) Refer patients with central causes of vertigo to the medical team, and patients with peripheral causes of vertigo to the ENT team.

FACIAL NERVE PALSY

DIAGNOSIS

(1) Upper motor neurone paralysis:
- (i) There is weakness of the lower facial muscles, often associated with other neurological signs such as hemiplegia.
- (ii) The cause is usually a stroke.

(2) Lower motor neurone paralysis:
- (i) There is weakness of the whole side of the face including the forehead muscles.
- (ii) Causes include:
  - (a) Bell's palsy with an abrupt onset sometimes associated with postauricular pain;

(b) Trauma to the temporal bone or a facial laceration in the parotid area;

(c) Tumours such as an acoustic neuroma or parotid malignancy;

(d) Infection such as acute otitis media, chronic otitis media with cholesteatoma or geniculate herpes zoster, the Ramsay Hunt syndrome;

(e) Miscellaneous including Guillain–Barré syndrome, sarcoidosis, diabetes.

(3) Examination must therefore include assessment of the external auditory canal, eardrum, parotid region and a full neurological examination.

MANAGEMENT

(1) Refer all acute cases with associated signs immediately to the medical, surgical or ENT team according to the likely aetiology.

(2) Give prednisolone 50 mg orally daily to a patient with Bell's palsy if seen within 2 days of onset and refer to the next ENT clinic.

TRAUMATIC CONDITIONS OF THE NOSE

FRACTURED NOSE

DIAGNOSIS

(1) This injury is usually obvious following a direct blow causing swelling, deformity and epistaxis.

(2) Exclude a more serious facial bone fracture, e.g. with CSF rhinorrhoea from cribriform plate damage (see page 337).

(3) Look carefully for a septal haematoma, which will lead to necrosis of the nasal cartilage and septal collapse if it is not drained.

(i) The nasal passage is blocked by a dull-red swelling replacing the septum, associated with marked nasal obstruction.

MANAGEMENT

(1) Refer a grossly deformed or compound fracture to the ENT team, as well as any patient with a septal haematoma. Refer more serious facial bone fractures to the maxillofacial surgery team.

(2) Otherwise, refer the patient to the ENT clinic within the next 5 days if operative treatment to straighten the nose for cosmetic reasons is requested.

(3) Do *not* take an x-ray as this will not alter the clinical management.

FOREIGN BODY IN THE NOSE

DIAGNOSIS AND MANAGEMENT

(1) This may be quite asymptomatic or lead to a serosanguinous, offensive, unilateral nasal discharge.

(2) If the object is easily accessible in the anterior part of the nose, attempt removal with a bent hook or pair of forceps.

(3) However (as with the foreign body in the ear), if removal is difficult, or a child is uncooperative, refer immediately to the ENT team. Sudden posterior dislodgement with inhalation of the foreign body is a real danger.

NONTRAUMATIC CONDITIONS OF THE NOSE

EPISTAXIS

DIAGNOSIS

(1) This is usually spontaneous in children, occurring from vessels in Little's area on the anterior part of the septum, possibly precipitated by rhinitis or minor trauma (e.g. nose picking).

(2) In adults the bleeding occurs posterior to Little's area and may be associated with hypertension or a bleeding diathesis, including anticoagulant drugs.

(3) In the elderly bleeding occurs high in the posterior part of the nose from arteriosclerotic vessels, and rapidly leads to haemorrhagic shock if profuse.

MANAGEMENT

(1) Bleeding from Little's area:

  (i)   Pinch the anterior part of the nose for 10 min with the patient sitting forwards until the bleeding stops. Then forbid the patient to pick, blow or sniff through the nose to prevent recurrence of the epistaxis.

  (ii) If a bleeding point persists, identify it with suction or by swabbing and anaesthetise the area with a cotton-wool pledget soaked in 4% lignocaine with adrenaline or in 5% cocaine (see below for maximum recommended dosage).

  (iii) Then cauterise the bleeding point with a silver nitrate stick touched onto the area for 10 s. Avoid overzealous application or cauterising both sides of the septum, as this will lead to septal necrosis.

(2) Persistent anterior bleeding and failed cautery:

  (i)   Anterior nasal pack.

    (a) Cover the patient and yourself with protective drapes and wear a face mask and goggles.

    (b) Apply local anaesthetic with cotton-wool pledgets soaked in either 4% lignocaine with adrenaline (maximum dose 12 ml or approximately 500 mg lignocaine in a 65-kg patient, i.e. 7 mg/kg), or 5% cocaine (maximum dose 2 ml or 100 mg in a 65-kg patient, i.e. 1.5 mg/kg).

    (c) Use 2.5 cm BIPP-impregnated gauze (BIPP = bismuth and iodoform paraffin paste) or a calcium alginate (Kaltostat) 2 g pack.

    (d) Insert successive horizontal layers, introduced along the floor of the nose using Tilley's nasal dressing forceps.

     (e) Remember in the adult that the nose extends 6.5–7.5 cm backwards to the posterior choanae (see Fig. 12).

(ii)   Anterior nasal tamponade.

Balloon catheters or nasal tampons are available as an alternative to packing. They are much easier to insert although are more expensive.

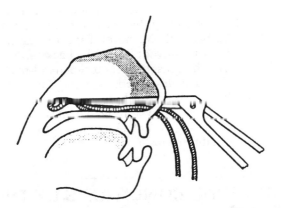

(a)

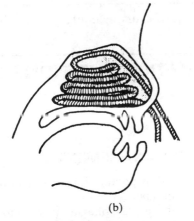

(b)

Fig. 12. (a) Anterior nasal packing, introducing the first loop along the floor of the nose and building upwards. (b) The pack in place.

(iii)   Refer the patient to the ENT team for admission and removal of the pack within 48 h.
(3) Severe posterior bleeding:
    (i)   Send blood for FBC, clotting study and G&S. Establish an intravenous infusion before the patient becomes hypotensive, and restore the circulation.
    (ii)   Attempt to stem posterior nasal bleeding by inserting a Foley urethral catheter far back along the floor of the nose, inflate the retaining balloon with air, and pull the catheter forwards to occlude the back of the nose. Tape the catheter to the cheek to prevent it slipping backwards.
       (a)   Then insert an anterior nasal pack as previously described.
       (b)   Occasionally both sides of the nose require packing to stop the bleeding.
    (iii)   Refer the patient immediately to the ENT team for admission.

TRAUMATIC CONDITIONS OF THE THROAT

See under 'Neck injuries: airway injury' on page 147.

NONTRAUMATIC CONDITIONS OF THE THROAT

TONSILLITIS

DIAGNOSIS AND MANAGEMENT

(1) This is either viral or bacterial, usually due to the beta-haemolytic streptococcus.
(2) There is sore throat, dysphagia, fever and foetor. A febrile convulsion may be precipitated in a child under 5 years old.

(3) Clinically it is impossible to distinguish a viral from a bacterial cause. Remember that glandular fever may present with a grey, exudative tonsillitis.

(4) Give the patient penicillin V 250 mg orally q.d.s. for 10 days and an antipyretic analgesic such as paracetamol. Return the patient to their general practitioner.

PERITONSILLAR ABSCESS (QUINSY)

DIAGNOSIS AND MANAGEMENT

(1) This may follow tonsillitis and is more common in adults.

(2) There is a worsening of the illness with high temperature, muffled voice, dysphagia referred earache and trismus.

(3) Examination shows unilateral swelling of the soft palate, with displacement of the tonsil downwards and medially and deviation of the uvula to the unaffected side.

(4) If difficulty in breathing supervenes, particularly in children, consider whether this could be epiglottitis and manage accordingly (see page 280).

(5) Otherwise refer the patient immediately to the ENT team for operative drainage. Give benzylpenicillin 1 Mu (600 mg) i.v. q.d.s.

FOREIGN BODY IN THE PHARYNX

DIAGNOSIS

(1) Fish or meat bones are the commonest objects to cause symptoms.

(2) Usually a fish bone will impact in the tonsil, base of the tongue, or posterior pharyngeal wall and may be seen by depressing the tongue to visualise the tonsil, or using a laryngeal mirror to see the back of the tongue and posterior pharynx.

(3) If no bone is seen despite symptoms, request a lateral soft-tissue x-ray of the neck. Calcification in the hyoid, thyroid, cricoid and laryngeal cartilages may cause confusion.

MANAGEMENT

(1) Attempt to remove the fish bone from the tonsil or the back of the tongue using Tilley's curved forceps.

   (i)   If this fails in a patient with pain or salivating excessively, refer the patient immediately to the ENT team.

   (ii)   Occasionally the pharyngeal mucosa has only been scratched, and if symptoms are minimal, prescribe an antibiotic such as amoxycillin 500 mg orally t.d.s., and ask the patient to return in 24 h for review.

(2) Refer the patient immediately to the ENT team for oesophagoscopy, if oesophageal impaction with dysphagia, excessive salivation, local tenderness or retrosternal pain is suspected (see below).

SWALLOWED FOREIGN BODY

DIAGNOSIS

(1) Coins are the commonest objects swallowed by preschool children, although small children swallow almost anything and the elderly may swallow their dentures.

(2) Oesophageal impaction, usually around the cricopharyngeus at the level of C6 is suggested by dysphagia, excessive salivation, local tenderness or retrosternal pain, but may be totally asymptomatic.[1]

(3) Button batteries pose a particular risk as they may cause local mucosal erosion and toxicity from mercury release.

(4) Occasionally airway obstruction occurs from upper oesophageal impaction or the object may in fact have been inhaled not swallowed (see page 280).

MANAGEMENT

(1) Request x-rays of the neck and chest to look for oesophageal impaction:

   (i)   Include PA and lateral views both to avoid missing a radio-opaque object superimposed over the skeletal or cardiac shadows on the PA view, and to differentiate tracheal lodgement.

(ii)   An abdominal x-ray is only indicated for button-battery ingestion, or for symptoms such as abdominal pain, distension or gastrointestinal bleeding.

(2) Refer the following patients immediately to the ENT team:

(i)   Airway obstruction or foreign body inhalation;
(ii)   Oesophageal impaction suspected clinically;
(iii)   Oesophageal lodgement seen on x-ray or inferred from prevertebral soft-tissue swelling, soft-tissue gas or air in the upper oesophagus;
(iv)   Button battery seen in the oesophagus or stomach.

(3) Otherwise, if the patient is asymptomatic and neck and chest x-rays are normal, allow the patient home:

(i)   Reassure the parents that most objects will pass spontaneously;
(ii)   Request immediate review if symptoms develop;
(iii)   Consider a repeat abdominal x-ray after 4 days in button battery ingestion if it has not been passed in the stools.
(iv)   Otherwise, repeat x-rays are only required if the patient develops symptoms.

STRIDOR

See page 279 in the paediatric section.

REFFRENCE

1   Cooke M.W., Glucksman E.E. (1991). Swallowed coins. *British Medical Journal*; **302**:1607.

OPHTHALMIC EMERGENCIES

Ophthalmic emergencies may be conveniently grouped into traumatic or nontraumatic, then subdivided further according to whether the eye is red, painful or has diminished visual acuity.

VISUAL ACUITY

(1) Visual acuity must always be recorded, with distance glasses if they are worn, at the start of every eye examination before any drops or dyes have been introduced.
   (i)   Acuity is measured by reading a Snellen chart at a distance of 6 m.
   (ii)   Each eye is tested separately and the lowest line that can be read accurately is recorded. 6/6 is normal vision.
(2) Ask patients with refractive errors who have left their glasses at home to look through a pinhole, to optimise their visual acuity.

TOPICAL OPHTHALMIC PREPARATIONS

The following preparations are indicated when referred to in the text.
(1) Antibiotic drops: 0.5% chloramphenicol solution, 2 drops 2 to 3-hourly.
(2) Antibiotic ointment: 1% chloramphenicol ointment, one application to the lower lid conjunctival sac 4-hourly, or at night (if eye drops are used during the day).
(3) Local anaesthetic: 1% amethocaine solution or 0.4% oxybuprocaine solution, 1 or more drops as required. (The patient must then wear a protective eye pad for 1–2 h until corneal sensitivity returns.)
(4) Fluorescein corneal stain: fluorescein sodium strips, or 2% fluorescein solution (do not use with soft contact lenses).
(5) Short-acting mydriatic dilating drops to examine the fundus: 1% tropicamide, 2 drops repeated after 15 min if

necessary (do not use in patients with narrow anterior chambers to avoid precipitating glaucoma).

(6) Miotic to constrict the pupil or reverse a mydriatic: 2% pilocarpine 1 or 2 drops.

Note: steroid preparations should *not* be used except by an experienced ophthalmologist. Any condition diagnosed that needs treatment with steroid drops also requires an ophthalmic opinion first.[1]

TRAUMATIC CONDITIONS OF THE EYE

PERIORBITAL HAEMATOMA (BLACK EYE)

DIAGNOSIS AND MANAGEMENT

(1) This is caused by a direct blow. If bilateral, suspect local trauma to the nose or a basal skull fracture (see page 130).

(2) Always make the following assessment:

    (i) Check that the patient can see, if necessary by opening the eyelids manually. Test visual acuity using distance glasses if they are worn, or a pinhole aperture if they are unavailable.

    (ii) Check the eyeball for damage. Examine the cornea for abrasions, the anterior chamber for hyphaema, and the pupil size and reactions. Also check for the presence of a red reflex through the pupil and a normal fundus.

    (iii) Refer any abnormal findings suggestive of one of the above complications immediately to the ophthalmology team.

    (iv) Test that the eye movements are full and the eyeball is not tethered, suggesting a 'blow-out' fracture of the orbital floor (see page 336).

    (v) Feel that the bony margin of the orbit is intact.

        (a) If a 'blow out' or a malar fracture is suspected, request appropriate facial x-rays and refer the patient to the maxillofacial surgery team.

(3) Otherwise, give the patient an analgesic such as para-cetamol 500 mg and codeine phosphate 8 mg (co-codamol), and chloramphenicol eye ointment if the eye is shut.

(4) Review the patient within 48 h when the swelling has decreased to confirm the absence of significant ocular damage.

SUBCONJUNCTIVAL HAEMATOMA

DIAGNOSIS AND MANAGEMENT

Two types are recognised, spontaneous and traumatic.

(1) *Spontaneous*:
   (i)   This may arise from coughing or from atherosclerotic vessels, particularly in the elderly, and is occasionally associated with hypertension or a bleeding diathesis.
   (ii) Check the blood pressure and reassure the patient that the blood will disperse within 2 weeks. No treatment is needed.

(2) *Traumatic*:
   (i)   This may be due to a surface conjunctival foreign body, a penetrating foreign body or a scleral perforation. Gentle digital assessment may reveal reduced eyeball tone in penetration of the globe.
   (ii) Refer all patients with a suspected serious cause as above immediately to the ophthalmology team.
   (iii) If the posterior margin cannot be seen, this suggests a basal skull fracture. In this case, refer the patient to the surgical team (see page 130).

EYELID LACERATION

DIAGNOSIS AND MANAGEMENT

(1) If the laceration involves the tarsal plate, the upper eyelid, the lid margin or the medial canthus and the

lacrimal apparatus, refer the patient directly to the ophthalmology or plastic surgery team.

(2) Otherwise, suture the eyelid under local anaesthesia using fine 6/0 synthetic monofilament sutures, which are removed by 4 days.

EYELID BURN

DIAGNOSIS AND MANAGEMENT

(1) The eye must be carefully examined for evidence of corneal or scleral damage before oedema makes the examination impossible, although the blink reflex usually protects the globe.

(2) Give the patient antibiotic drops, analgesia and tetanus prophylaxis, and refer immediately to the ophthalmology team.

CHEMICAL BURNS TO THE EYE

DIAGNOSIS AND MANAGEMENT

(1) Alkalis are far more dangerous than acids, and include common agents such as cement, plaster powder, oven and drain cleaner.

(2) The mainstay of treatment is immediate, copious, prolonged irrigation with normal saline from an intravenous giving set. Local anaesthetic drops may initially be needed to open the eye.

(3) Take care to irrigate all corners of the eye and to evert the upper eyelids to remove any particulate matter and to irrigate the superior fornix of the conjunctiva.

(4) Refer the patient immediately to the ophthalmology team, unless fluorescein staining reveals no corneal damage and the surrounding conjunctiva appears normal and is pain free.

(5) Provide adequate analgesia if necessary with morphine 5 mg i.v. plus an antiemetic such as metoclopramide 10 mg i.v.

CONJUNCTIVAL FOREIGN BODY

DIAGNOSIS AND MANAGEMENT

(1) Usually a piece of grit blows in the eye causing pain, redness and watering.

(2) The object is easily seen by direct vision and is removed with a moistened cotton-wool bud after instilling local anaesthetic. An eye pad is then worn for 1–2 h until the return of normal sensation.

(3) If the object impacts on the upper subtarsal conjunctiva, nothing will be seen immediately but the eye will be red and painful to blink. Fluorescein staining will reveal linear corneal abrasions.

(4) Evert the upper eyelid:

    (i)   Stand behind the patient to evert the upper lid, supporting the head against your body.

    (ii)   Instruct the patient to look downwards, pull the upper lid eyelashes down and then up and over the tarsal plate, which is held depressed by a glass rod or orange stick (see Fig. 13).

    (iii) Remove the foreign body with a moistened cotton-wool bud.

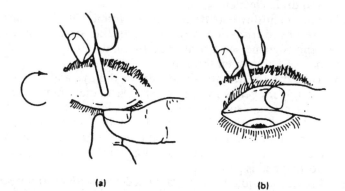

(a)   (b)

Fig. 13. (a) Eversion of the upper eyelid. (b) Demonstrating the subtarsal conjunctiva.

(5) Always stain the cornea with fluorescein for evidence of corneal abrasion; if it is present give the patient antibiotic drops for 2 days.

(6) Remember the possibility of intraocular penetration, e.g. by a metal fragment (see page 320).

CORNEAL FOREIGN BODY

DIAGNOSIS AND MANAGEMENT

(1) The foreign body may be obvious, or revealed by fluorescein staining.

(2) Instil local anaesthetic drops and attempt removal of the foreign body with a moistened cotton-wool bud or the edge of a hypodermic needle, introduced from the side.

(3) However, deep or recalcitrant foreign bodies and those with extensive rust rings should be left alone. Refer the patient to the ophthalmology team to avoid causing further damage on attempted removal.

(4) If local anaesthetic was used, pad the eye for 1–2 h until the return of normal sensation. Treat any residual corneal epithelial defect demonstrated with fluorescein as for a corneal abrasion (see below).

(5) Review the patient within 2 days to exclude infection. If there is evidence of an infected corneal ulcer refer the patient immediately to the ophthalmology team.

CORNEAL ABRASION

DIAGNOSIS AND MANAGEMENT

(1) Corneal abrasion is due to a foreign body or to direct injury from a finger, stick or a piece of paper.

(2) There is intense pain, watering and blepharospasm. Local anaesthetic drops may be needed before the eye can be opened properly.

(3) Fluorescein staining will reveal the damage. Give the patient 0.5% chloramphenicol eye drops, mydriatic drops and review within 2 days. An eye pad is no longer recommended.[2]

(4) The cornea should be fully healed by then, but if there is delayed healing or a recurrence, refer the patient to the ophthalmology team.

FLASH BURN (ARC EYE)

DIAGNOSIS AND MANAGEMENT

(1) A superficial keratitis that occurs after exposure to ultraviolet light, from welding without using protective goggles, or from a sun lamp.
(2) There is pain, watering and blepharospasm occurring after a few hours. Fluorescein staining reveals a pitted corneal surface.
(3) Instil local anaesthetic drops, mydriatic drops and double-pad the eyes until the return of normal sensation and the blepharospasm settles. Give an analgesic such as paracetamol 500 mg and codeine phosphate 8 mg (co-codamol).
(4) Recovery occurs within 12–24 h.

BLUNT TRAUMA TO THE EYE

DIAGNOSIS AND MANAGEMENT

(1) Injury to the eye should always be considered in any trauma to the face. It must not be forgotten when other injuries appear more dramatic, or periorbital oedema obscures the eye.
(2) Blunt trauma may cause a sequence of injuries from the front to the back of the eye:
  (i)   Periorbital haematoma or subconjunctival haemorrhage.
  (ii)   Corneal abrasion or laceration.
  (iii) Bleeding into the anterior chamber, called hyphaema. This may be microscopic or macroscopic with formation of a fluid level.
  (iv)   A fixed pupil or torn iris, known as traumatic mydriasis and iridodialysis respectively.

(v)   A dislocated lens or subsequent traumatic cataract.

(vi) Vitreous haemorrhage causing a dull or absent red reflex and obscuring the fundus.

(vii) A retinal tear, with retinal detachment seen as a dark, wrinkled, ballooned area diametrically opposite any resultant visual field defect.

(viii) Retinal oedema (*commotio retinae*) seen as whitish areas of oedema, usually associated with haemorrhage.

(ix) Optic nerve damage, causing blindness with no direct pupillary response to light.

(x)   Ruptured globe with marked visual loss, a soft eye and shallow anterior chamber.

(xi) Orbital fracture, usually a 'blow-out' fracture of the orbital floor (see page 336)

(3) All these conditions require immediate examination by the ophthalmology team. The patient must not be allowed home in the meantime but should lie quietly semi-upright pending expert assessment:

(i)   Ideally pad both eyes and give appropriate analgesia;

(ii) Protect a suspected ruptured globe with an eye shield, not a pad.

PENETRATING TRAUMA TO THE EYE

DIAGNOSIS AND MANAGEMENT

(1) Penetrating trauma is usually obvious, although on occasions it may initially be extremely difficult to recognise.

(2) The following injuries are possible:

(i)   Corneal laceration often with prolapse of the iris into the defect.

(ii) Scleral perforation with chemosis or local haemorrhage. This must be differentiated from a trivial subconjunctival bleed.

(iii) Collapse of the anterior chamber, hyphaema or vitreous haemorrhage, pupil irregularity and lens dislocation.

(3) *Intraocular foreign body*:
  (i)   This is usually a metal fragment from using a hammer and chisel, metal drill or grinding wheel.
  (ii) Sudden sharp pain is followed by localised redness, or the outside of the eye may appear normal and the incident forgotten.
  (iii) Carefully examine for a puncture wound and use an ophthalmoscope to inspect the inner eye, although a traumatic cataract may preclude this.
  (iv) Always x-ray the orbit in all suspected cases if there is the remotest possibility of penetration. Two soft-tissue films, with the eye looking up and down, should identify a radiodense intraocular foreign body.
(4) Instil antibiotic eye drops (*not* ointment), protect the eye from further damage with an eye shield and give tetanus prophylaxis.
  (i)   Provide analgesia if required, e.g. morphine 5 mg i.v. with an antiemetic metoclopramide 10 mg i.v.
  (ii) Give gentamicin 80 mg i.v. plus ceftriaxone 1 g i.v.
(5) Refer all cases of documented penetrating injury to the eye and actual or suspected intraocular foreign bodies immediately to the ophthalmology team.

CONDITIONS AFFECTING THE EYELIDS

BLEPHARITIS

DIAGNOSIS AND MANAGEMENT

(1) Blepharitis is an infection of the eyelid margin, causing red, itchy, crusted lids, which may become chronic with an allergic element. Styes and chalazions are commonly associated.
(2) Prescribe antibiotic ointment, but refer the patient to the ophthalmology clinic for follow-up if this condition becomes persistent or recurrent.

EXTERNAL STYE (HORDEOLUM)

DIAGNOSIS AND MANAGEMENT

(1) This is due to an infection of a lash follicle pointing on the lid margin.
(2) Give the patient antibiotic ointment and remove any protruding eyelash. Warm bathing may help.

INTERNAL STYE

DIAGNOSIS AND MANAGEMENT

(1) This is an infected Meibomian gland within the tarsal plate. It does not discharge as easily as an external stye and may leave a residual Meibomian cyst. Alternatively it may point and discharge inwards through the tarsal plate, causing conjunctivitis and discharge.
(2) Refer the patient to the ophthalmology clinic before it discharges inwards. Warm bathing is unhelpful.

MEIBOMIAN CYST (CHALAZION)

DIAGNOSIS AND MANAGEMENT

(1) This feels like a hard pip within the tarsal plate.
(2) Refer the patient to the ophthalmology clinic for incision and curettage.

DACRYOCYSTITIS

DIAGNOSIS AND MANAGEMENT

(1) Dacryocystitis is inflammation of the lacrimal sac in the inner canthus of the lower eyelid (dacryoadenitis is inflammation of the lacrimal gland in the outer upper eyelid).
(2) There is a localised, tender, red swelling and watering of the eye due to the blocked lacrimal duct.
(3) Start a systemic antibiotic such as flucloxacillin 500 mg orally q.d.s. after sending a swab of any exuding pus.
(4) Refer the patient to the next ophthalmology clinic.

ORBITAL CELLULITIS

DIAGNOSIS AND MANAGEMENT

(1) This condition follows sinusitis or a periorbital injury, with intense pain, swelling and protrusion of the eye.

(2) There is generalised malaise, a raised temperature and a discharging, congested eye with ophthalmoplegia. Adjacent sinuses are tender when involved in the infection.

(3) Take blood cultures and give flucloxacillin 1 g i.v. and ceftriaxone 1 g i.v.

(4) Refer the patient immediately to the ophthalmology team and obtain an ENT opinion if the paranasal sinuses are involved.

(5) Complications particularly in children can occur within hours, including meningitis, central retinal vein occlusion, optic nerve compression and cavernous sinus thrombosis.

BASAL CELL CARCINOMA (RODENT ULCER)

DIAGNOSIS AND MANAGEMENT

(1) Basal cell carcinoma is the commonest malignancy of the eyelid, more frequent on the lower lid and following prolonged exposure to sunlight.

(2) An early, opalescent pink papule with surface telangiectasia progresses slowly to an ulcerated nodule with a pearly, rounded edge that is locally invasive.

(3) Refer the patient to the next ophthalmology clinic for treatment by either excision, curettage, cryotherapy or radiotherapy in the elderly.

HERPES ZOSTER OPHTHALMICUS (OPHTHALMIC SHINGLES)

DIAGNOSIS AND MANAGEMENT

(1) This presents as a vesicular rash over the distribution of the ophthalmic division of the trigeminal (fifth) cranial nerve. Pain and tingling often precede the rash.

(2) The patient is usually unwell and in pain. The eye may be affected resulting in blepharitis, conjunctivitis, keratitis, uveitis, secondary glaucoma, ophthalmoplegia or optic neuritis.

(3) Treatment of the varied ocular problems is awkward as eyelid swelling makes topical therapy difficult, and pain may be incapacitating.

(4) Therefore refer the patient to the ophthalmology team for inpatient care.

    (i)   Acyclovir 800 mg orally 5 times daily with 3% acyclovir ophthalmic ointment decreases pain, corneal damage and uveitis.

THE PAINFUL, RED EYE

There are five important causes to consider:
(1) acute conjunctivitis;
(2) acute episcleritis and scleritis;
(3) acute keratitis;
(4) acute iritis;
(5) acute glaucoma.

ACUTE CONJUNCTIVITIS

DIAGNOSIS

(1) The causes are:
    (i)   allergic;
    (ii)   bacterial, such as staphylococci, pneumococci, gonococci or *Haemophilus*;
    (iii) viral, particularly adenovirus or enterovirus;
    (iv) chlamydial.

(2) There is generalised conjunctival injection with gritty discomfort, mild photophobia and variable discharge. Vision should be normal.

MANAGEMENT

(1) Clean away the discharge with moist cotton-wool balls, and avoid irritating cosmetics or eye lotions.

(2) Allergic conjunctivitis responds to steroid drops, but these must only be prescribed by an ophthalmologist. Initially prevent secondary bacterial infection with antibiotic drops and refer the patient to the ophthalmology clinic.

(3) Bacterial conjunctivitis requires frequent antibiotic drops, as often as hourly in severe cases, and ointment at night. Refer the patient to the ophthalmology clinic if the infection does not settle.

(4) Viral conjunctivitis, due to the adenovirus or enterovirus, is highly contagious and person-to-person spread is rapid, unless scrupulous care is taken with hand washing.

    (i)   Give antibiotic drops and ointment to prevent secondary bacterial infection.

    (ii)   Refer the patient to the next ophthalmology clinic for a definitive diagnosis and to monitor for the development of keratitis.

(5) Chlamydial conjunctivitis usually occurs in young adults causing chronic bilateral conjunctivitis with mucopurulent discharge. The cornea may be involved (keratitis).

    (i)   The diagnosis is difficult but should be suspected when conventional antibiotic therapy fails.

    (ii)   Associated urethritis or salpingitis may suggest the aetiology.

    (iii)   Special swabs and treatment with topical and oral tetracycline are best discussed with the Special Clinic (genitourinary medicine clinic).

ACUTE EPISCLERITIS AND SCLERITIS

DIAGNOSIS

(1) Episcleritis is localised inflammation beneath the conjunctiva adjacent to the sclera. Scleritis is a more painful localised inflammation of the sclera itself. Rheumatoid arthritis may be associated.

(2) The eye is locally red and sore with reflex watering but no discharge. Progression to eyeball perforation occurs in scleritis.

MANAGEMENT

(1) Send blood for FBC, ESR and rheumatoid factor and commence a nonsteroidal anti-inflammatory agent such as diclofenac (Voltarol) 50 mg orally t.d.s.
(2) Refer the patient to the ophthalmology team for definitive treatment including steroid eye drops.

ACUTE KERATITIS

DIAGNOSIS

(1) This is inflammation of the cornea due to many possible causes, including viruses such as herpes simplex and the adenovirus, bacterial infection of a corneal ulcer, abrasion, exposure or contact-lens wear.
(2) The main distinguishing feature from conjunctivitis is the prominent pain, with diminution of vision if there is a central ulcer or a hypopyon (pus in the anterior chamber).
(3) Fluorescein staining will demonstrate a marginal or central ulcer. Where herpes simplex is implicated the ulcer is typically branching or dendritic.

MANAGEMENT

(1) Steroid eye drops are absolutely forbidden.
(2) Commence antibiotic drops and refer the patient immediately to the ophthalmology team.

ACUTE IRITIS

DIAGNOSIS

(1) This is occasionally due to exogenous infection from a perforating wound or corneal ulcer.
(2) Otherwise ill-understood endogenous mechanisms linked with HLA-B27 and seronegative arthropathy are involved as in ankylosing spondylitis, Reiter's syndrome, ulcerative colitis, Crohn's disease and Still's

disease. Other causes include sarcoidosis, toxoplasmosis, TB, syphilis and herpes zoster ophthalmicus.

(3) There is circumcorneal ciliary injection, constant pain, photophobia and impaired vision. The pupil contracts and tiny aggregates of cells may be seen on the inner surface of the cornea, known as keratic precipitates.

(4) In severe cases pus forms in the anterior chamber causing a hypopyon, and the iris may adhere to the anterior lens surface causing posterior synechiae.

MANAGEMENT

(1) Refer the patient immediately to the ophthalmology team for treatment with steroid drops and cycloplegics.

(2) Attacks may become recurrent and progress to secondary glaucoma.

ACUTE GLAUCOMA

DIAGNOSIS

(1) Glaucoma is associated with a narrowed anterior chamber with obstruction to the outflow of aqueous humour.

(2) It is more common in middle-aged or elderly hypermetropes (long-sighted people) and is precipitated by pupillary dilatation.

(3) There is severe throbbing, boring pain accompanied by nausea, vomiting and prostration. Vision is reduced with haloes around lights and the cornea becomes hazy with a fixed, semidilated oval pupil. On gentle palpation the eye feels hard.

MANAGEMENT

This is an ocular emergency requiring urgent referral to the ophthalmology team. On their advice commence:

(1) Miotic drops such as pilocarpine every 5 min for up to 1 h;

(2) Acetazolamide 500 mg orally or slowly intravenously;

(3) An antiemetic such as metoclopramide 10 mg i.v. and analgesia such as morphine up to 2.5 mg i.v. for severe pain.

SUDDEN LOSS OF VISION IN THE UNINFLAMED EYE

Conditions to be considered include:
(1) central retinal artery occlusion;
(2) central retinal vein occlusion;
(3) vitreous haemorrhage;
(4) retinal detachment;
(5) optic neuritis.

CENTRAL RETINAL ARTERY OCCLUSION

DIAGNOSIS

(1) This condition is most common in the elderly arteriosclerotic patient, but it may occur due to emboli or in association with temporal arteritis.
(2) There is sudden blindness associated with a relative afferent pupillary defect (Marcus Gunn pupil):
    (i)   A swinging light directed into one eye, then briskly into the other produces apparent dilatation of the pupil in the affected eye, as the relaxing consensual reflex in the good eye is dominant.
    (ii) It is a reliable sign of a unilateral or asymmetrical optic nerve or retinal lesion.
(3) The fundus is milky white, the optic disc pale and swollen and a cherry-red spot develops at the macula in 1–2 days.

MANAGEMENT

(1) Refer the patient urgently to the ophthalmology team, as treatment within 1–2 h may restore the circulation.
(2) Gentle ocular massage may help, and rebreathing into a paper bag to dilate the retinal vessels by CO_2 retention.

(3) If there is a prodromal history of headache, scalp tenderness and malaise consider temporal arteritis.

    (i)   Measure an ESR and if raised, give the patient prednisolone 60 mg orally to prevent the other eye being involved (see page 60).

CENTRAL RETINAL VEIN OCCLUSION

DIAGNOSIS

(1) This condition is most common in elderly patients with atherosclerosis, hypertension and simple glaucoma. Diabetes and hyperviscosity also predispose.

(2) Visual loss is less abrupt but may be noticed suddenly. A relative afferent pupillary defect may be seen in severe cases.

(3) The fundus shows congested veins with scattered flame haemorrhages and optic disc swelling.

MANAGEMENT

(1) There is no specific treatment although predisposing conditions must be looked for.

(2) Refer the patient to the ophthalmology clinic to monitor for the development of secondary acute glaucoma (some weeks later) from neovascularisation.

VITREOUS HAEMORRHAGE

DIAGNOSIS

(1) This may be traumatic or spontaneous, associated with diabetes, various blood disorders and retinal detachment.

(2) There is a reduced or absent red reflex and diminution in vision, preceded by floaters.

MANAGEMENT

(1) Refer the patient to the ophthalmology team to exclude retinal detachment and to look for other predisposing conditions.

(2) Vitrectomy may be necessary if the haemorrhage fails to clear.

RETINAL DETACHMENT

DIAGNOSIS

(1) This may be traumatic, or spontaneous in myopes (short-sighted people) or follow a vitreous haemorrhage.
(2) There is peripheral visual loss, like a curtain, that may be profound if the macula is affected. A preceding history of floaters or sudden flashing lights is common.
(3) The retina is dark, wrinkled and ballooned, and the choroid may be seen as a red tear. A relative afferent pupil defect is seen if the detachment is large.

MANAGEMENT

Refer the patient immediately to the ophthalmology team for possible surgical repair.

OPTIC NEURITIS

DIAGNOSIS

(1) This may be idiopathic, post-viral or associated with demyelination from multiple sclerosis.
(2) There is loss of central vision with pain on moving the eye, and a relative afferent pupillary defect (see page 327).
(3) If the optic disc is involved, there is papillitis that must be distinguished from papilloedema:
   (i)   Papilloedema tends to to be bilateral, pain-free with normal pupil responses. There is no visual loss but an enlarged blind-spot is found on field testing.

MANAGEMENT

(1) Examine the patient for other signs of demyelination, but never inform him or her of your suspicions at this early stage.

(2) Refer the patient to the ophthalmology clinic.

REFERENCES

1   Lavin M. J., Rose G. E. (1986). Use of steroid eye drops in general practice. *British Medical Journal*; **292**:1448–50.

2   Easty D.L. (1993). Is an eye pad needed in cases of corneal abrasion? *British Medical Journal*; **307**:1022.

MAXILLOFACIAL AND DENTAL EMERGENCIES

TRAUMATIC CONDITIONS OF THE FACE AND MOUTH

LACERATIONS

MANAGEMENT

(1) *Face*: meticulously debride facial cuts under local anaesthesia and suture using fine 5/0 synthetic monofilament nylon (Ethilon) sutures, removed by 4 days.

(2) *Lips*:
- (i) Use 3/0 or 4/0 absorbable sutures such as polyglactin (Vicryl) for intraoral lesions and 5/0 synthetic monofilament nylon sutures for external lacerations.
- (ii) If the full thickness of the lip is lacerated vertically, breaching the vermilion border, refer the patient to the oral surgery team to avoid subsequent cosmetic deformity from inexperienced repair.

(3) *Tongue*:
- (i) Most lacerations may be left unless large and through the edge, or bleeding profusely, when an absorbable suture such as 3/0 catgut or polyglactin (Vicryl) is used.
- (ii) Advise a regular mouthwash of warm saline within 24 h.

TOOTH INJURIES

MANAGEMENT

(1) *Chipped tooth*:
- (i) Enamel or dentine damage: The tooth will be sensitive but viable. Advise the patient to avoid hot or cold drinks and refer to the patient's own dentist.
- (ii) Pulp space exposed: The tooth may be bleeding from the pulp, and sensitive to light touch. Refer the patient immediately to the oral surgery team, as there is a risk of pulp infection or necrosis.

(2) *Displaced tooth*:
  (i)   Do not manipulate unless the tooth is about to fall out, when it should be firmly replaced in its socket.
  (ii) Refer the patient to a dental surgeon as soon as possible for immobilisation of the tooth.

(3) *Avulsed permanent incisor tooth*:
Reposition of a dry, avulsed tooth within 30 min outside its socket or up to 2 h if stored in saliva or milk gives the best chance of successful reimplantation:
  (i)   If immediate reimplantation is not performed, transport the tooth in the buccal sulcus of the patient's own cheek, or in milk if the patient is uncooperative or unconscious.
  (ii) On arrival in the A&E department, handle the tooth by the crown only, rinse it in saline and replace back into the socket with firm pressure. No analgesia is necessary.
  (iii) Splint the tooth with aluminium foil, give the patient an antibiotic such as amoxycillin 500 mg orally t.d.s. and tetanus prophylaxis.
  (iv) Refer the patient to a dental surgeon as soon as possible.

Note: if a tooth or denture is actually missing following trauma, perform a PA and lateral CXR to exclude inhalation into the lung or PA and lateral neck x-rays if obstruction in the upper oesophagus is suspected (see page 308).

(4) *Bleeding tooth socket*:
  (i)   This can be post-traumatic or post-extraction.
  (ii) Clear out clots and arrest haemorrhage using a calcium alginate (Kaltostat) dressing or gauze roll.
  (iii) If the bleeding persists, attempt to close the mucosa over the socket using 3/0 absorbable polyglactin (Vicryl) sutures after infiltrating with 1% lignocaine with 1 in 200 000 adrenaline. If this fails, refer the patient to the oral surgery team.

(5) *Broken dentures*: always save these as they will be invaluable to the maxillofacial surgeon to aid in the fixation of jaw fractures or if a splint is needed.

FRACTURED MANDIBLE

DIAGNOSIS

(1) This injury is due to a blow on the jaw causing a unilateral or frequently bilateral fracture. Occasionally the temporomandibular joint may be dislocated or the condylar process driven back into the temporal bone, causing bleeding and deformity of the external auditory canal.

(2) There is localised pain, particularly on attempted jaw movement and malocclusion. Inside the mouth, bruising or bleeding of the gum and discontinuity of the teeth occur if there is a displaced fracture.

(3) There will be numbness of the lower lip if the inferior dental nerve has been damaged in its course through the mandible.

(4) X-rays should include an AP view, with a panoramic OPG (orthopantomogram) or lateral views of the mandible.

MANAGEMENT

(1) Clear the airway of any clots or debris and ensure that the tongue or a portion of the mandible does not slip back and occlude the pharynx.

(2) Refer any unstable or grossly displaced injuries immediately to the maxillofacial surgery team.

(3) Otherwise, for an undisplaced fracture give the patient tetanus prophylaxis and antibiotics, as most fractures are compound into the mouth. Use co-amoxiclav 500/125 (amoxycillin 500 mg and clavulanic acid 125 mg) one tablet orally t.d.s. for 5 days.

(4) Refer the patient to the next maxillofacial surgery clinic.

DISLOCATED MANDIBLE

DIAGNOSIS

(1) Dislocation may occur spontaneously after yawning or follow a blow to the jaw. It may be unilateral or bilateral and may become recurrent.

(2) The mouth is stuck open and is painful.

(3) Exclude drug-induced dystonia due to metoclopramide or phenothiazines by direct questioning, as this may mimic or even predispose to dislocation. It is treated with benztropine (Cogentin) 1–2 mg i.v.

MANAGEMENT

(1) Request an AP and lateral x-ray of the temporo-mandibular joints to exclude an associated fracture, unless the dislocation was spontaneous or recurrent.

(2) In the absence of a fracture, try to reduce without sedation. If unsuccessful, use intravenous midazolam 2.5–5 mg with full resuscitation facilities available.

   (i)   Stand in front of the patient and press firmly downwards by applying pressure with your thumbs inside the mouth to the angle of the jaw to distract the condyle, placing your fingers under the chin. Then push backwards to relocate the condyle in the fossa.

   (ii) Repeat the x-ray to confirm reduction and refer to the next maxillofacial surgery clinic. Advise the patient to avoid excessive mouth opening.

   (iii) Apply a barrel bandage to discourage wide opening, if the dislocation is recurrent, or required intravenous midazolam.

FRACTURE OF THE ZYGOMATIC OR MALAR COMPLEX

DIAGNOSIS

(1) This injury is due to a direct blow to the cheek which may fracture the zygomatic arch in isolation, but more usually causes a 'tripod' fracture through three structures:

   (i)   superiorly through the zygomaticofrontal suture;
   (ii) laterally through the zygomatic arch;
   (iii) medially through the zygomaticomaxillary suture or the infraorbital foramen.

(2) There is flattening of the malar process best seen from above (which may be masked by oedema), epistaxis, subconjunctival haemorrhage extending posteriorly, and infraorbital nerve paraesthesia. Jaw movement may be limited if the coronoid process obstructs under the zygomatic arch.

(3) Although these fractures are best diagnosed clinically, particularly by finding local bony tenderness, request facial x-rays including occipitomental views (OM 10° and OM 30°):

    (i) Look carefully for the fractures comparing with the normal side;

    (ii) Or look for secondary evidence of injury, e.g. opacity of the maxillary antrum from bleeding into the maxillary sinus or overlying soft-tissue swelling.

MANAGEMENT

(1) Advise the patient not to blow his or her nose as subcutaneous emphysema may occur if the paranasal sinuses are involved.

(2) Commence amoxycillin 500 mg orally t.d.s. (or erythromycin 500 mg orally q.d.s. if the patient is allergic) as most fractures are compound into the maxillary sinus, and an analgesic such as paracetamol 500 mg and codeine phosphate 8 mg (co-codamol).

(3) Refer the patient to the maxillofacial surgery team within 24 h for elevation of the depressed cheekbone within 7 days.

'BLOW OUT' FRACTURE OF THE ORBITAL FLOOR

DIAGNOSIS

(1) This uncommon fracture is due to blunt trauma to the eye from a small object the size of a squash ball, driving the eyeball backwards and rupturing the weak bony floor of the orbit. Orbital fat and occasionally the inferior rectus muscle herniate through the defect into the maxillary sinus.

(2) It is essential to initially exclude blunt trauma to the eye (see page 318). The fracture itself causes enophthalmos that may be masked by periorbital oedema, infraorbital nerve loss and diplopia with restricted upwards gaze due to trapping of the inferior rectus muscle.

(3) Facial x-ray often fails to show the fracture but it can be inferred from an opaque maxillary sinus or a fluid level from the bleeding, and a 'tear drop' soft-tissue opacity hanging from the roof of the sinus.

MANAGEMENT

(1) Refer blunt eye damage immediately to the ophthalmology team.

(2) Commence amoxycillin 500 mg orally t.d.s. and 1% chloramphenicol eye ointment 4-hourly.

(3) Refer the patient to the maxillofacial surgery team within 24 h.

MIDDLE THIRD OF FACE FRACTURES

DIAGNOSIS

(1) These complicated fractures are usually bilateral and are divided into three eponymous groups:

  (i) Le Fort I:
    (a) This is due to a blow to the maxilla causing a horizontal fracture separating the alveolar bone and teeth from the maxilla.
    (b) There is epistaxis and malocclusion, and crepitus may be elicited.

  (ii) Le Fort II:
    (a) This is a pyramidal fracture extending up from a Le Fort I fracture to involve the nasal skeleton and the middle of the face. The middle of the face is thus 'stove in', elongating the face and causing malocclusion.
    (b) The airway may be compromised and CSF may leak from the nose.

    (iii) Le Fort III:
           (a) This dislocates the entire midfacial skeleton
               from the base of the skull (craniofacial
               dysjunction).
           (b) There is massive facial swelling and bruising,
               and often brisk pharyngeal bleeding that may
               cause haemorrhagic shock. The airway is
               again in danger.

MANAGEMENT

(1) Attend urgently to the airway:
    (i)   Sometimes, if the face is stove in, the whole
          segment may be lifted forwards manually to
          relieve the airway.
    (ii) Otherwise, orotracheal intubation or even
          cricothyrotomy are required if there is difficulty
          maintaining an adequate airway.
(2) Remember that the direct force to the face may have
    caused an additional cervical spine injury or head injury.
    (i)   Lateral cervical spine x-ray and a head CT scan
          are therefore the priority.
    (ii) Specific facial view x-rays must wait until all the
          other major injuries are stabilised and a cervical
          spine injury is excluded.
(3) Refer all fractures immediately to the maxillofacial
    surgery team.

NONTRAUMATIC CONDITIONS OF THE MOUTH

TOOTHACHE

DIAGNOSIS AND MANAGEMENT

(1) Toothache is usually due to inflammation of the pulp
    space in a carious tooth.

(2) Exclude a dental abscess (see below) and give the patient an analgesic such as paracetamol 500 mg and codeine phosphate 8 mg (co-codamol). Return the patient to his or her own dentist.

DENTAL ABSCESS

DIAGNOSIS AND MANAGEMENT

(1) An apical or periapical abscess is an extension of a pulp space infection.
   (i)   The tooth is tender to tapping, with associated soft-tissue swelling and continuous pain.
   (ii) There may be systemic malaise and fever.
(2) If the patient is severely ill, or the abscess is pointing extraorally, refer to the oral surgery team.
(3) Otherwise, commence an antibiotic such as amoxycillin 500 mg orally t.d.s., give an analgesic (e.g. codeine phosphate 30–60 mg orally q.d.s.), and return the patient to his or her own dentist.

LUDWIG'S ANGINA

DIAGNOSIS AND MANAGEMENT

(1) This condition is a bilateral, fulminant, brawny cellulitis of the sublingual and submandibular areas, associated with poor dental hygiene or dental instrumentation.
(2) There is trismus, dysphagia, submandibular pain and swelling and a risk of sudden respiratory obstruction.
(3) Admit the patient immediately under the ENT team for careful observation of the airway and give benzylpenicillin 3 Mu (1.8 g) i.v.

SUBMANDIBULAR SWELLINGS

DIAGNOSIS AND MANAGEMENT

(1) Several causes are possible:
   (i)   *Submandibular stone*. This intermittently blocks the submandibular duct, causing pain and swelling

aggravated by food. The stone is palpable on bimanual examination and is seen on x-ray. Refer the patient to the oral surgery team.

(ii) *Submandibular abscess*. The pain is constant with associated malaise, swelling in the angle of the jaw and trismus. Refer the patient to the oral surgery team.

(iii) *Mumps*. This usually affects the parotids and is usually bilateral, but can affect the submandibular glands. Remember the association with orchitis.
    (a) Give patients paracetamol elixir and reassure them.

(iv) *Dental abscess*. This may point downwards from a molar tooth to the submandibular area.

(v) *Lymph node enlargement*. The commonest causes of cervical adenopathy in this area are tonsillitis and pharyngitis.

(vi) *Rare causes*. These include carcinoma, lymphoma, sarcoid, TB or a bony swelling.

GYNAECOLOGICAL EMERGENCIES

VAGINAL EXAMINATION

(1) Most gynaecological emergencies that present with abdominal pain or vaginal bleeding will require the opinion of the gynaecology team, who should be asked to perform the vaginal examination if the A&E doctor is inexperienced.

(2) However, in every case still make a detailed history and examination, send urgent blood samples to the laboratory and institute resuscitative procedures as necessary. Also consider possible nongynaecological conditions.

PRESCRIBING IN PREGNANCY

(1) The British National Formulary (BNF) includes an appendix at the end, containing a table of drugs that can have harmful effects on the fetus during pregnancy, and indicates the trimester of risk.

(2) Ideally all drugs should be avoided in the first trimester.

(3) Therefore, it is essential to enquire as to the possibility of pregnancy in every female of reproductive age.

(4) This is also relevant when requesting x-rays, although most hospital radiology departments have their own guidelines to minimise the risk of irradiation in early pregnancy.

(5) The BNF also has another appendix containing a table of drugs excreted in breast milk to be avoided.

GYNAECOLOGICAL CAUSES OF ACUTE ABDOMINAL PAIN

The following conditions may present with acute abdominal pain:

(1) ruptured ectopic pregnancy;
(2) acute salpingitis;
(3) ruptured ovarian cyst;

(4) torsion of an ovarian tumour;
(5) endometriosis.

RUPTURED ECTOPIC PREGNANCY

DIAGNOSIS

(1) Ectopic pregnancy is more common in patients with previous pelvic inflammatory disease or tubal surgery, and in patients using the intrauterine contraceptive device (IUCD).
(2) Ectopic pregnancy usually presents from 6 to 12 weeks of pregnancy. Patients presenting early may not realise they are pregnant, although there may be breast tenderness, nausea or a history of recent unprotected intercourse.
    (i) It must always be considered in every patient with menstrual irregularities, vaginal bleeding or lower abdominal pain.
(3) The unstable form presents with sudden abdominal pain, often referred to the shoulder tip, followed by scanty vaginal bleeding, proceeding to circulatory collapse and haemorrhagic shock.
(4) The stable form has a prodromal history of lower abdominal pain and slight vaginal bleeding that is typically dark brown ('prune juice'), although the bleeding can be fresh red.
(5) Examination in the unstable form reveals a pale, collapsed, hypotensive patient with a tender, rigid, silent abdomen.
(6) In the stable form, there is localised lower abdominal tenderness and guarding to one side, with discomfort and swelling in that lateral fornix on vaginal examination, and a smaller uterus than expected for the duration of amenorrhoea.

MANAGEMENT

(1) *Unstable ectopic*:
    (i) Give the patient oxygen, insert a large-bore intravenous cannula, send blood for FBC, U&E, blood sugar and cross-match 4 units of blood.

(ii)   Commence an infusion of crystalloid such as normal saline or colloid such as polygeline (Haemaccel) and refer the patient immediately to the gynaecology team. Inform theatre and the duty anaesthetist.

(2) *Stable ectopic*:

(i)   Insert an intravenous cannula and send blood for FBC, U&E, blood sugar and G&S. Send serum for a pregnancy test if a urinary test kit is unavailable (see below).

(ii)   Perform a pregnancy test:

(a)   A serum radioimmunoassay pregnancy test for beta-HCG in blood is extremely sensitive, with a negative test ruling out a recent ectopic or abortion, although it takes time to do and may not be available after hours.

(b)   Alternatively, use a urinary beta-HCG monoclonal antibody immunoassay. This can be done rapidly in the A&E department and may be positive even before the first missed period. Again a negative test virtually rules out an ectopic.

(iii)   Request a transabdominal ultrasound scan to demonstrate a gestation sac within the uterus, which effectively excludes an ectopic. A transvaginal ultrasound scan is even more sensitive as it identifies signs of the extrauterine pregnancy itself.

(iv)   Refer all cases to the gynaecology team. Ultimately a laparoscopy or laparotomy confirms the condition and allows definitive management.

(v)   Give rhesus-negative mothers anti-D immunoglobulin 250 units i.m. to prevent maternal formation of antibodies from isoimmunisation.

ACUTE SALPINGITIS

DIAGNOSIS

(1) This is a sexually transmitted disease caused principally by chlamydial or gonococcal infection. Recurrent infections are increasingly likely to cause infertility.

(2) It presents acutely with fever, malaise, bilateral lower abdominal pain, dyspareunia, menstrual irregularities and vaginal discharge.

(3) These is a temperature on examination with bilateral lower abdominal tenderness and guarding. On vaginal examination pain and warmth in each lateral fornix, with pain on moving the cervix, are elicited. This is known as a positive cervical excitation test.

(4) The white blood cell count is raised, and a serum or urine beta-HCG pregnancy test is negative.

MANAGEMENT

(1) Send blood for FBC, blood culture and send an MSU. Perform a pregnancy test.

(2) Remove an IUCD if it is present and send it for culture.

(3) Send an endocervical and urethral swab for gonococcal culture in a suitable transport medium such as Stuart's, and an endocervical swab for chlamydia, if this service is available.

(4) Refer all patients who are unwell, unable to rest at home, pregnant (unusual) or in whom the diagnosis is uncertain to the gynaecology team.

(5) In the remainder, commence doxycycline 100 mg orally b.d. and metronidazole 400 mg orally b.d. (avoiding alcohol), both for 2 weeks.

(6) Review the patient in the next gynaecology clinic or refer her to the genitourinary medicine Special Clinic for follow-up.

(7) Advise abstinence from sexual intercourse until the partner has also been seen and treated in a Special Clinic.

RUPTURED OVARIAN CYST

DIAGNOSIS AND MANAGEMENT

(1) There is sudden, moderate, lower abdominal and pelvic pain without gastrointestinal symptoms.

(2) The patient is afebrile with localised tenderness, but no mass is felt. A pregnancy test is negative.

(3) Refer the patient to the gynaecology team.

TORSION OF AN OVARIAN TUMOUR

DIAGNOSIS AND MANAGEMENT

(1) Fibroids or cysts that twist, or suddenly distend from a bleed cause sudden lower abdominal pain, often with preceding episodes of milder pain.

(2) The patient may have nausea, a low-grade fever and localised abdominal tenderness with a palpable mass.

(3) Send blood for FBC, collect an MSU and exclude pregnancy with a pregnancy test. Refer the patient to the gynaecology team. Pelvic ultrasound or laparoscopy may be required to confirm the diagnosis.

ENDOMETRIOSIS

DIAGNOSIS AND MANAGEMENT

(1) There is a preceding history of recurrent abdominal and flank pain, worse at the time of menstruation and immediately following the period, dyspareunia, painful defaecation, infertility and acquired dysmenorrhoea.

(2) This is a difficult diagnosis requiring the opinion of the gynaecology team.

BLEEDING IN EARLY PREGNANCY

Two important causes are ectopic pregnancy and spontaneous abortion. Induced septic abortion is now rare.

Spontaneous abortion is the expulsion of the products of conception before the 28th week of pregnancy. In practice this presents as vaginal bleeding or abdominal pain.

Note: refer any bleeding or abdominal pain in a patient over 18 weeks pregnant directly to the labour ward (this rule may differ from hospital to hospital).

SPONTANEOUS ABORTION

DIAGNOSIS

There are five recognised stages of spontaneous abortion:
(1) *Threatened abortion*:
- (i) This is commonest up to 14 weeks gestation, causing mild cramps and transient vaginal bleeding.
- (ii) The uterine size is compatible with the duration of pregnancy. A guide to the expected size of the uterus is given by:
  - (a) Bimanual examination: the uterus is the size of a hen's egg at 7 weeks; an orange at 10 weeks; a grapefruit at 12 weeks.
  - (b) Abdominal palpation: the fundus reaches the symphysis pubis at 12 weeks and the umbilicus at 24 weeks.
- (iii) The external cervical os is closed on speculum examination.

(2) *Inevitable abortion*:
- (i) The bleeding is heavier, followed by cramps that are more persistent.
- (ii) The external cervical os is open 0.5 cm or more and the products of conception may be found in the vagina or protruding from the cervical canal.
- (iii) The symptoms and signs of pregnancy will disappear. These include amenorrhoea, nausea, vomiting, breast enlargement, tenderness, tingling and areolar pigmentation and frequency of micturition.

(3) *Incomplete abortion*:
- (i) Bleeding remains heavy and the cramps persist with the passage of clots and the products of conception.
- (ii) These may be found on examination or have been previously noted by the patient.

(4) *Complete abortion*: the bleeding and cramps stop after the conceptus has been passed and the signs of pregnancy disappear.

(5) *Missed abortion*:

   (i)   The products of conception are retained, although cramps and bleeding are replaced by a brownish vaginal discharge.

   (ii) The uterus is small and irregular, and ultrasound fails to detect fetal heart motion.

   (iii) Infection and disseminated intravascular coagulation may occur.

MANAGEMENT

(1) Send blood for FBC and G&S if the bleeding is heavy and commence an infusion of normal saline. Confirm recent pregnancy with a serum or urine beta-HCG immunoassay pregnancy test.

(2) Remove the products of conception with sponge forceps if they are blocking the cervical canal, to help relieve pain, bradycardia and hypotension. Send them for histology to exclude a hydatidiform mole.

(3) Refer all patients to the gynaecology team for bed rest (threatened abortion), or evacuation of retained products of conception (ERPC) for inevitable or incomplete abortion.

(4) Remember all rhesus-negative mothers must be given anti-D immunoglobulin 500 units i.m. within 72 h, to prevent maternal formation of antibodies to fetal rhesus-positive cells.

INDUCED SEPTIC ABORTION

DIAGNOSIS AND MANAGEMENT

(1) This is usually the result of criminal abortion (a felony in England since 1861) or occasionally therapeutic abortion, legalised in England in 1967 in certain well-defined circumstances.

(2) There is rapidly spreading pelvic infection with salpingitis, peritonitis, septic pelvic and pulmonary thrombophlebitis, leading to septicaemic shock and death.
(3) The patient is unwell with fever, abdominal pain, foul vaginal discharge and bleeding, leading to hypotension, oliguria, confusion, then coma.
(4) Give the patient oxygen, start an intravenous infusion and send blood for FBC, coagulation profile, U&E, blood sugar and blood culture.
(5) Commence benzylpenicillin 3 Mu (1.8 g) i.v., gentamicin 80 mg i.v. and metronidazole 500 mg i.v. and refer her urgently to the gynaecology team for evacuation of the uterine contents or emergency hysterectomy.

CONDITIONS IN LATE PREGNANCY

Ideally all patients over 18 weeks pregnant should be sent straight to the labour ward. Occasionally they are too ill or there is not time to get them there. Thus the following conditions may be seen, all requiring prompt request for obstetric help.

CONFUSING TERMINOLOGY

Two confusing terms are used in obstetric practice:
(1) *Gravida*. This is the number of pregnancies of any gestation including the current pregnancy, with twins counting as one.
(2) *Parity*.
  (i)   This is the number of previous pregnancies of 28 weeks or more whether live or stillborn. Distinction is made between events after and before 28 weeks.
  (ii) It is described as 'para $x + y$', where x is deliveries after 28 weeks, whether stillborn or live with twins counting as two, and y is pregnancies ending before 28 weeks, whether by spontaneous or therapeutic abortion.

ANTEPARTUM HAEMORRHAGE

DIAGNOSIS AND MANAGEMENT

(1) Vaginal bleeding after 28 weeks pregnancy is a life-threatening emergency when due to placenta praevia or placental abruption.

(2) *Never* examine the patient vaginally or with a speculum for fear of precipitating torrential vaginal haemorrhage.

(3) Give oxygen, place the patient in the left lateral position and start an intravenous infusion if the patient is hypotensive or shocked. Send blood for FBC, coagulation profile and cross-match 4 units.

(4) Refer the patient immediately to the obstetric team.

PRE-ECLAMPSIA AND ECLAMPSIA

DIAGNOSIS AND MANAGEMENT

(1) Pre-eclampsia is diagnosed on finding oedema, proteinuria and hypertension with a systolic blood pressure over 140 mmHg and a diastolic over 90 mmHg in the third trimester of pregnancy (or greater than a 25 mmHg systolic rise or 15 mmHg diastolic rise compared with early pregnancy).

(2) If pre-eclampsia becomes fulminating there is headache, visual symptoms, nausea, vomiting and abdominal pain. Irritability and hyper-reflexia may herald generalised eclamptic convulsions. Oliguria and disseminated intravascular coagulation are common.

(3) Call the obstetric team urgently. Give oxygen, gain venous access and send blood for FBC, coagulation profile, U&E, LFTs and uric acid.

    (i)   Control fits with magnesium sulphate 4 g i.v. over 5 min, followed by an infusion at 1 g/h. This now appears to be the drug of choice.[1]

        (a) An alternative regime is diazepam (Diazemuls) 5–10 mg i.v. followed by phenytoin

15 mg/kg by infusion. Take the advice of the obstetric team.

(ii) Initiate BP control with hydralazine 5 mg i.v. slowly.

EMERGENCY DELIVERY

MANAGEMENT

(1) Call the obstetric team and paediatric or neonatal team immediately.

(2) Allow the mother to lie or sit semi-upright and give her 50% nitrous oxide with oxygen (Entonox) during the first half of the contractions.

(3) A mediolateral episiotomy may be needed in primiparous women.

(4) Ask the mother to pant and thus to stop pushing as the head crowns, usually with the occiput upwards, which is followed by rotation (restitution) of the head.

(5) The next contraction delivers the anterior shoulder by gentle downward traction on the head, which is followed by the posterior shoulder and trunk.

(6) The baby is then delivered by lifting the head and trunk up and over the symphysis pubis, to lie on the mother's abdomen.

(7) Cut the cord immediately if it is wound tightly around the baby's neck; otherwise it is clamped off or tied with two 2/0 silk ties after delivery and divided.

(8) Aspirate mucus from the baby's nose and mouth and keep the baby warm by wrapping it in a blanket. Be prepared to intubate if there is apnoea.

(9) Leave the placenta to deliver itself; avoid the temptation to pull on the cord for fear of causing uterine inversion. Try gentle abdominal massage to stimulate a uterine contraction, or give syntocinon 5 units and ergometrine 0.5 mg (Syntometrine) 1 ml i.m. to prevent postpartum haemorrhage and aid delivery of the placenta.

(10) The mother can commence suckling her baby immediately; this will stimulate uterine contraction to help expel the placenta and reduce the risk of haemorrhage.

CARDIOPULMONARY RESUSCITATION IN LATE PREGNANCY

DIAGNOSIS

(1) Causes of cardiac arrest in late pregnancy include utero-placental bleeding, cerebrovascular haemorrhage, pulmonary embolus, amniotic fluid embolus and cardiac disease.

(2) Impaired venous return from inferior vena caval compression by the gravid uterus, with the patient supine, will render resuscitative efforts ineffective unless it is deliberately minimised.

MANAGEMENT

(1) Tilt the patient laterally using a wedge or pillow under the right side, and displace the uterus by lifting it manually upwards and to the left off the great vessels.

(2) Perform basic and advanced life support as for adult cardiac arrest (see page 2), but compared to the nonpregnant patient:
  (i) Intubation is more tricky due to large breasts, short neck, laryngeal oedema, etc;
  (ii) There is increased risk of regurgitation and pulmonary aspiration;
  (iii) Effective external chest compression is more difficult due to flared ribs, raised diaphragm, breast enlargement and inferior vena caval compression.

(3) Consider immediate caesarean section if the resuscitation is not rapidly successful, having called the obstetric and paediatric teams on the arrival of the patient:
  (i) Ideally surgical intervention should be within 5 min of cardiac arrest for optimum maternal and neonatal survival.[2]
  (ii) Continue cardiopulmonary resuscitation throughout the procedure and afterwards until a stable rhythm with a sustained cardiac output is obtained.

TRAUMA IN PREGNANCY

The best treatment for the fetus is to rapidly stabilise the mother. Treatment priorities for trauma in a pregnant patient are the same as for the nonpregnant patient.

MANAGEMENT

(1) Follow the immediate management guidelines as for multiple injuries (see page 135), but note the following additional considerations:

    (i)   Tilt the supine patient laterally using a wedge or pillow under the right hip and manually displace the gravid uterus upwards and to the left, to minimise impaired venous return from inferior vena caval compression in the third trimester.

    (ii)   Protect the airway from the increased risk of gastric regurgitation and pulmonary aspiration.

    (iii)   Larger amounts of blood may be lost before obvious signs of hypovolaemia such as tachycardia, hypotension and tachypnoea occur, as both maternal blood volume and cardiac output increase in pregnancy.

    (iv)   Fetal distress without necessarily signs of maternal shock occurs readily, as blood is shunted preferentially away from the uterus to maintain the maternal circulation following blood loss.

    (v)   Perform peritoneal lavage when indicated, using a supraumbilical approach with the minilaparotomy technique, after first inserting a nasogastric tube and urethral catheter.

    (vi)   Retroperitoneal bleeding with pelvic fracture after blunt trauma may be massive from the engorged pelvic veins.

(2) After initial resuscitation of the patient, assess the fetus during the secondary survey including fundal height, uterine tenderness, contractions, fetal movement and fetal heart rate. Use a fetal stethoscope or Doppler ultrasound for the heart rate:

    (i)   Fetal distress is indicated by:

(a) bradycardia less than 110 beats per minute (normal 120–160 beats per minute);

(b) loss of fetal heart acceleration to fetal movement or late deceleration after uterine contractions.

(ii) Important causes of fetal distress or fetal death in trauma include maternal hypovolaemia, placental abruption and uterine rupture:

(a) signs of placental abruption vary from vaginal bleeding, abdominal pain, tenderness, increasing fundal height and premature contractions to maternal shock;

(b) signs of traumatic uterine rupture, which occurs more commonly in the second half of pregnancy, range from abdominal pain to maternal shock or a separately palpable uterus and fetus.

(iii) Arrange continuous fetal monitoring e.g. by cardiotocography for a minimum of 6 h, even after apparently minor maternal trauma.

(iv) Give all rhesus-negative mothers anti-D immunoglobulin 500 units i.m.

(3) Therefore, call the obstetric team to review and admit *all* pregnant trauma cases. Call the paediatric team in addition if the fetus is over 26–28 weeks gestation and immediate delivery is indicated.

(i) Emergency caesarean section performed within 5 min of maternal cardiac arrest maximises the chance of fetal survival and may also improve maternal outcome.

POSTCOITAL CONTRACEPTION

Occasionally patients present for emergency contraceptive measures after unprotected intercourse. There are two possibilities:

(1) Postcoital pill. This may be used up to 72 h after unprotected intercourse.

(2) Intrauterine contraceptive device. This may be used within 5 days after unprotected intercourse. Refer the patient to the family planning clinic or specialist pregnancy advice service for this.

POSTCOITAL PILL

MANAGEMENT

(1) Use 100 µg ethinyloestradiol and 500 µg levonorgestrel contained in 2 tablets of Ovran, or in 2 of the tablets of Schering PC4, a commercially prepared package which includes a comprehensive explanatory leaflet.

(2) The 2 tablets are given followed exactly 12 h later by a further two. If vomiting occurs within 3 h of the first dose, give a repeat prescription with an antiemetic.

(3) Never use this method when absolute contraindications to oestrogens are present such as crescendo angina, transient ischaemic attacks, liver disease, a history of thromboembolism and undiagnosed genital tract bleeding.

(4) Warn the patient that her next period may be early or late and advise the use of a barrier contraceptive device until then.

(5) Refer all patients for follow-up to their general practitioner or a family planning clinic to check that:
  (i)   the pregnancy test is negative 3–4 weeks later;
  (ii) there is no ectopic pregnancy (slight increased risk if the method fails);
  (iii) the patient receives proper contraceptive advice for the future.

MISSED ORAL CONTRACEPTIVE PILL

Usually a frantic call on the telephone requests advice on what to do following a missed oral contraceptive pill.

(1) If the patient is on the combined oral contraceptive:
  (i)   *Up to 12 h late*:
        (a) Take the missed pill and carry on as usual.

(ii)   *Over 12 h late*:
    (a)   Continue normal pill taking, but for the next 7 days either abstain from sex or use an alternative method of contraception such as the sheath.
    (b)   If these 7 days run beyond the end of the packet, start the next packet immediately the present one is over, i.e. no gap between packets.
    (c)   This will mean that no period may occur until the end of two packets, but this is not dangerous.
    (d)   If everyday (ED) pills are being used, miss out the seven inactive pills.
    (e)   Remember that missing a pill at the beginning or end of a cycle is potentially more critical than missing one in the middle.

(2) If the patient is on the progestogen-only pill:
    (i)   *Over 3 h late*:
        (a)   Continue normal pill taking but abstain from sex or use an alternative method of contraception for the next 7 days.

DOMESTIC VIOLENCE

DIAGNOSIS

(1) Most victims are women, although a similar management approach is applicable to both sexes.
(2) Domestic violence affects women of every class, race and religion. It may commence at times of acute stress such as unemployment or first pregnancy.
(3) The victim may present with injury, abdominal pain, substance abuse, attempted suicide, rape or with multiple somatic complaints.
(4) Victims may attend late, be evasive and embarrassed or their partner may answer for them.

MANAGEMENT

(1) Ensure privacy by interviewing alone without the partner. Ask gently but directly about the possibility of violence, which may initially be denied.

(2) Record all injuries measuring bruises or lacerations with a ruler and institute any urgent treatment to save life.

(3) Enquire about any additional risk of physical or sexual abuse to other members of the household, particularly children (see page 274).

(4) Offer admission if it is unsafe for the patient to return home or if acute psychiatric illness is present, e.g. depression.

(5) Call the duty social worker. However, if in the meantime the patient wishes to return home, give written contact numbers including:
   (i)   general practitioner;
   (ii)   social worker;
   (iii) local police;
   (iv)   Women's Aid: National Helpline:
          Telephone (Bristol) 0117 963 3542.

RAPE

Follow a standard procedure in all cases of alleged rape in which the patient requests or accepts police involvement.

MANAGEMENT

(1) Be accompanied by a senior female nurse escort at all times.

(2) Record a careful history of exactly what occurred and when, and a description of the assailant.

(3) Examine the patient for associated injuries, measuring bruises or lacerations with a ruler. Request informed, written consent to keep all clothing for forensic analysis.

(i)   Then undress the patient on a sheet to collect any debris.

(ii)   Wrap each garment in a brown paper bag fastened with tape and labelled with the patient's name, the date, nature of sample and person taking the sample.

(4) Institute any urgent treatment to save life, e.g. cross-match and starting a transfusion for haemorrhage.

(5) Contact the police to inform the duty police surgeon, who will perform the forensic examination aimed at collecting evidence regarding:

(i)   proof of sexual contact;

(ii)   lack of consent;

(iii)   identification of the assailant.

(6) Request a senior gynaecology doctor to perform the examination of the external genitalia and vagina, if the duty police surgeon is unavailable.

(7) The police will also try to arrange for a designated sexual offences unit to attend, usually nonuniformed women police officers who have received special training.

(8) Call the duty social worker or give the patient written contact telephone numbers/addresses if a social worker is not immediately available.

(9) Offer admission to all patients and discuss the following issues:

(i)   the need for the postcoital pill to prevent pregnancy;

(ii)   the need to exclude a sexually transmitted disease by attending a genitourinary medicine Special Clinic in the next few days;

(iii)   specialist counselling from various external organisations, e.g. the Rape Crisis Centre in London:

    (a) telephone 0171 837 1600 for 24-h counselling;

    (b) telephone 0171 278 3956 for their head office recorded information.

(iv)   aftercare instructions with details of all the tests performed, treatments provided and other arrangements made.

REFERENCES

1   The Eclampsia Trial Collaborative Group (1995). Which anticonvulsant for women with eclampsia? Evidence from the Collaborative Eclampsia Trial. *Lancet*; **345**:1455–1463.

2   Oates S., Williams G.L., Rees G.A.D. (1988). Cardiopulmonary resuscitation in late pregnancy. *British Medical Journal*; **297**: 404–405.

References

PSYCHIATRIC EMERGENCIES

DELIBERATE SELF-HARM

DIAGNOSIS

(1) The most common method of deliberate self-harm is by acute poisoning.
   - (i) This may be freely admitted, or be evident from finding a suicide note or an empty bottle beside the patient.
   - (ii) The possibility should also be considered in any unconscious or confused patient, or in patients with unexplained metabolic, respiratory or cardiac problems (see page 63).
(2) Other methods of deliberate self-harm include cutting the wrists or throat, shooting, hanging, drowning, gassing or jumping from a height.

MANAGEMENT

(1) Perform the necessary investigations and resuscitative procedures to save life and refer the patient directly to the medical, surgical or orthopaedic team if there is serious illness or injury.
(2) A medically unimportant acute poisoning, including a patient intoxicated with alcohol, may have been a serious self-harm attempt and should still be admitted for 24 h, possibly to the department's own observation ward.
(3) A full assessment may then be made the next day to decide on the further management of the patient.
   - (i) Assessment of suicidal intent. Enquire specifically about:
     - (a) present suicidal thoughts;
     - (b) previous deliberate self-harm;
     - (c) evidence of a premeditated act without the intention of being found.
   - (ii) Consider other high-risk factors including:
     - (a) mental illness, including depression and schizophrenia;

      (b) violent self-harm attempt, such as jumping, hanging or shooting;

      (c) chronic alcohol abuse or drug dependency;

      (d) older, single, urban, lonely male;

      (e) puerperium.

  (iii) Refer any patients considered to have a continuing suicide risk immediately to the psychiatric team.

  (iv) Make a psychiatric outpatient appointment for less acute problems and refer problems with a domestic or social basis to the social work team.

(4) In all cases, inform the general practitioner by telephone and by letter if the patient has been allowed home (preferably accompanied by a relative or friend).

THE CONFUSED PATIENT

'Confusion' should be reserved to describe a state of clouding of consciousness or disturbed awareness, which may fluctuate.

DIAGNOSIS

(1) There is a wide spectrum of confusional states between the following two extremes:

    (i) difficulty maintaining attention, irritability, emotional lability and illusions;

    (ii) delirium: disorientation in time and place, impaired memory, restlessness, hallucinations and poor comprehension.

(2) *Causes of confusion.*

    (i) Drugs:

      (a) intoxication or withdrawal from alcohol, LSD, cocaine and amphetamines;

      (b) side-effects (especially in the elderly) of analgesics, anticonvulsants, psychotropic, anticholinergic and antiparkinsonian drugs such as benzhexol and levodopa.

(ii)   Hypoxia:
    (a)   after head injury or chest injury;
    (b)   chest infection, pulmonary embolus, cardiac failure;
    (c)   respiratory depression from drugs or muscle disorders, e.g. myasthenia gravis or muscular dystrophy.

(iii) Metabolic:
    (a)   renal, liver, respiratory and cardiac failure;
    (b)   vitamin deficiency, e.g. thiamine or B_{12};
    (c)   electrolyte imbalance such as hyponatraemia, hypernatraemia and hypercalcaemia;
    (d)   acute intermittent porphyria.

(iv)   Endocrine:
    (a)   hypoglycaemia or hyperglycaemia;
    (b)   thyrotoxicosis, myxoedema, Cushing's syndrome, steroids and Addison's disease.

(v)   Cerebral:
    (a)   trauma;
    (b)   postictal state, complex partial (temporal lobe) seizures;
    (c)   cerebrovascular accident, subarachnoid haemorrhage;
    (d)   meningitis, encephalitis;
    (e)   space-occupying lesion, e.g. tumour, abscess or haematoma;
    (f)   hypertensive encephalopathy;
    (g)   systemic lupus erythematosus.

(vi)   Other infections: e.g. biliary tract, urinary tract or malaria.

(vii) Constipation and urinary retention in the elderly.

MANAGEMENT

(1) A detailed history and examination will help build up a picture of which condition(s) is responsible.

(2) Always exclude hypoglycaemia, and perform some or all of the following investigations based on the suspected aetiology:
    (i)   FBC, coagulation profile;

     (ii)   U&E, blood sugar, drug screen, calcium, liver function tests, thyroid function tests;

     (iii)   arterial blood gases;

     (iv)   blood cultures, MSU;

     (v)   CXR, ECG;

     (vi)   CT scan;

     (vii) LP.

(3) Admit all patients under the appropriate specialist team. Avoid the temptation to simply sedate the confused patient, without looking carefully for the underlying cause.

THE VIOLENT PATIENT

DIAGNOSIS

(1) Most violence encountered by staff in the A & E department will be the result of alcohol intoxication, either by the patient or by their relatives or friends, who may be irritated and angry at having to wait if the department is busy.

(2) Other causes for violent behaviour:

     (i)   Hypoglycaemia (including as the patient recovers from a hypoglycaemic episode after intravenous dextrose administration), hypoxia.

     (ii)   Drugs, including amphetamines, LSD and cocaine.

     (iii) Withdrawal syndromes from alcohol or barbiturates.

     (iv) Postictal state.

     (v)   Mental illness, particularly mania and paranoid schizophrenia.

MANAGEMENT

(1) Explain what is happening at all times, reassure the patient and avoid confrontation. Never turn your back on a patient or allow them between you and the cubicle door.

(2) Initially attempt verbal restraint by defining acceptable and unacceptable behaviour and their likely consequences.

(3) If verbal restraint fails, consider physical restraint:
- (i) Call the police or security guards and await adequate numbers (ideally 4 or 5 persons).
- (ii) Never try to restrain a patient single-handed especially if he has a weapon.
- (iii) Conversely, never remove physical restraints until a full evaluation has been made and help is standing by.

(4) If chemical restraint is indicated give haloperidol or droperidol 5–10 mg i.m. or slowly i.v. This may be supplemented with midazolam 5 mg i.v. for more rapid control.
- (i) Such treatment may be given without consent under common law in an emergency, if the patient is a danger to others or himself.
- (ii) Every sedated patient must then be monitored in a resuscitation area until the risks of respiratory depression and hypotension have passed.

(5) Record full details of events in the notes and the necessary action taken.

(6) Admit the patient under the medical or psychiatric team if further treatment is indicated.

ALCOHOL-RELATED PROBLEMS

Alcohol is causally related to virtually all types of trauma including motor vehicle accidents, accidents in the home, deliberate self-harm, assaults, drownings, child abuse and even falls in the elderly.

MEASUREMENT OF ALCOHOL LEVEL

Various methods are available, including a breath test, a urine test or a blood level. This may not be available out of hours, therefore an approximate blood alcohol level may be derived by measuring the serum osmolality and using the following formula:

Approximate blood alcohol in mg%:

= 5 × (measured osmolality – calculated osmolality),

where calculated osmolality = 2(Na + K) + urea + glucose.

Units: measured osmolality in mosmol/kg; Na, K, urea, glucose in mmol/l.

Note: the British blood alcohol legal limit for driving is 80 mg%, although people have walked unaided with levels in excess of 600 mg%! However, intoxication is marked above a level of 150 mg%, and coma usually occurs above a level of 300 mg%.

THE PATIENT WITH AN ALTERED CONSCIOUS LEVEL SMELLING OF ALCOHOL

MANAGEMENT

Never assume that a confused, obtunded or unconscious patient smelling of alcohol is simply drunk until you have excluded all of the following:

(1) Hypoglycaemia:
  (i)   Check a blood sugar on all 'drunks' and give 50 ml of 50% dextrose if it is low.
  (ii) Occasionally this may precipitate worsening of the confusion. Suspect Wernicke's encephalopathy, a condition associated with alcohol abuse and malnutrition causing ataxia, nystagmus and bilateral lateral rectus palsy. This requires immediate thiamine 100 mg i.v.
(2) Head injury:
  (i)   Always remember the possibility of an extradural or subdural haematoma.
  (ii) Commence neurological observations and perform a CT head scan if confusion persists or there is a deteriorating conscious level (see page 131).
    (a) A skull x-ray may be useful in the absence of a CT scan, but even if normal does not exclude intracranial injury.

(3) A coincidental medical problem:
  (i)   Epileptic fit;
  (ii)   Acute poisoning;
  (iii)   Cerebral haemorrhage;
  (iv)   Meningitis, chest infection, etc;
  (v)   Hypothermia;
  (vi)   Rib fracture, wrist fracture, abdominal trauma.
(4) An acute medical condition prevalent in alcoholics:
  (i)   Aspiration or pneumococcal pneumonia, TB;
  (ii)   Gastrointestinal haemorrhage;
  (iii)   Pancreatitis;
  (iv)   Liver failure;
  (v)   Withdrawal fits or delirium tremens;
  (vi)   Cardiac arrhythmia, cardiomyopathy;
  (vii)   Hypokalaemia, hypomagnesaemia, hypocal-
          caemia;
  (viii) Lactic acidosis;
  (ix)   Wernicke's encephalopathy.
(5) Thus, many patients will require admission to exclude the
    above conditions. If in doubt, always admit for observation.

ALCOHOL WITHDRAWAL

This is caused by an absolute or relative decrease in the usual
intake of alcohol, through lack of funds or by detention in
hospital or by the police.

DIAGNOSIS AND MANAGEMENT

Two conditions are recognised: the alcohol withdrawal
syndrome, and the progression to delirium tremens.
  (1) *Alcohol withdrawal syndrome*:
    (i)   This is common occurring within 12 h of absti-
          nence and lasting a few days. It is characterised by
          agitation, irritability, fine tremor, sweats and
          tachycardia.
    (ii) Commence diazepam 10 mg orally 2–6 hourly or
          chlordiazepoxide 20 mg orally 6 hourly until the
          patient is comfortable, plus thiamine 100 mg i.v. or
          i.m. daily.

    (iii)   Control fits with intravenous diazepam (Diazemuls) 5–10 mg, after excluding hypoglycaemia.

    (iv)   Refer the patient to the medical team.

(2) *Delirium tremens*:

    (i)   This is uncommon occurring 72 h after abstinence; there is clouding of consciousness, terrifying hallucinations, gross tremor, autonomic hyperactivity with tachycardia, dilated pupils, fever, sweating, dehydration and grand mal fits that may be prolonged (status epilepticus).

    (ii)   Delirium tremens is a medical emergency. Give diazepam (Diazemuls) 5–10 mg i.v. for fits, and exclude other causes of status epilepticus such as head injury and meningitis (see page 51).

    (iii)   Replace fluid and electrolyte losses, avoiding excessive normal saline in liver failure. Give thiamine 100 mg i.v. daily.

    (iv)   Refer all patients immediately to the medical team.

Note: never dispense chlormethiazole (Heminevrin) capsules in the A&E department to take home. They are best reserved for inpatient detoxification programmes only.

PROBLEM DRINKING

MANAGEMENT

(1) Alcohol-dependent patients often request help to stop drinking.

    (i)   If there is actual suicidal depression or total inability to cope at home, refer the patient immediately to the psychiatric team.

    (ii)   Otherwise, refer the patient to the appropriate psychiatric clinic for outpatient assessment, or to the social work department.

    (iii)   Meanwhile, give the patient written details of local support organisations to contact, such as:

(a) Alcoholics Anonymous.
Telephone: (London) 0171 352 3001
Head Office: (York) 01904 644026.
(b) Al-Anon. This organisation provides help and advice for the family and friends of problem drinkers.
Telephone: (London) 0171 403 0888.
(2) Always write to the general practitioner to enlist his or her help and support.

DRUG DEPENDENCY AND DRUG ABUSE

DIAGNOSIS

(1) Patients may be seen who are dependent on or abuse the following classes of drugs:
    (i)   opiates;
    (ii)   barbiturates;
    (iii) benzodiazepines;
    (iv)   alcohol;
    (v)   chlormethiazole;
    (vi)   stimulants including amphetamines or cocaine;
    (vii) miscellaneous substances including cannabis, LSD and solvents.
(2) Abrupt withdrawal of some of these drugs causes acute symptoms:
    (i)   Opiate withdrawal causes restlessness, excitability, muscle cramps, diarrhoea, tachycardia and sweating, known as 'cold turkey'.
    (ii)   Barbiturate withdrawal causes hallucinations and epileptic fits.
    (iii) Benzodiazepine withdrawal causes a rebound increase in tension, anxiety and apprehension with anorexia and insomnia.
(3) The health departments of the UK have produced a report 'Drug Misuse and Dependence' containing guidelines on clinical management. It is available from HMSO bookshops or by telephoning 0171 873 9090.

OPIATE ABUSE

MANAGEMENT

(1) Patients may need referral to the medical team for acute poisoning, abscesses, septicaemia, bacterial endocarditis, hepatitis B, pneumonia and, increasingly, HIV infection.

(2) Otherwise, if a regular opiate user needs admission to the observation ward within the department perhaps following an orthopaedic or minor operative procedure:

    (i) Give salicylate or paracetamol for mild or moderate pain, and methadone orally or i.m. for severe pain.

    (ii) If signs of opiate withdrawal occur such as agitation, cramps, pupillary dilatation, tachycardia and sweating, give the patient diazepam 5–10 mg orally, repeated as required.

    (iii) If the patient demands a controlled drug, explain that it is actually an offence for a doctor to administer or authorise the supply of a drug of addiction, except in the treatment of an organic disease or injury, unless licensed to do so by the Home Secretary.

    (iv) Moreover, the Misuse of Drugs (Notification of and Supply to Addicts) Regulations 1973 also require the doctor to notify the Chief Medical Officer at the Home Office in writing within 7 days of attendance, details of a person who he considers to be, or has reasonable grounds to suspect is addicted to a controlled drug, unless that person has already been notified.

(3) Refer patients wishing to stop their habit and seeking help to:

    (i) A drug dependency clinic;

    (ii) A local drug dependency organisation such as Narcotics Anonymous, telephone 0171 351 6794;

    (iii) The social work department;

    (iv) The patient's own general practitioner.

BARBITURATE, BENZODIAZEPINE AND SOLVENT ABUSE

MANAGEMENT

(1) Patients who abuse these groups of drugs all require referral to specialist clinics to coordinate their withdrawal regime. Help and advice is available from:

    (i) Psychiatric outpatient clinics.

    (ii) A local drug dependency organisation. These include:

        (a) MIND
(National Association for Mental Health)
Telephone 0171 637 0741.
This organisation provides self-help groups for withdrawal from tranquillisers.

        (b) 'Re-Solv', Society for the Prevention of Solvent and Volatile Substance Abuse. Telephone 01785 817885.

    (iii) The social work department.

    (iv) The patient's own general practitioner.

COMPULSORY ADMISSION

It is rarely necessary to detain a patient against his or her will in the A & E department under the Mental Health Act 1983 (MHA). However, if a patient is suffering from a mental disorder, which is severe enough to endanger his or her own health or safety, or that of others, detention will be required. Always request the help and advice of the psychiatric team in such circumstances. It is unusual to have to act in their absence.

(1) *Section 2: Admission for assessment.*

    (i) This is a 28-day order.

    (ii) Application to the hospital may be made by the nearest relative (as defined in section 26 of the MHA), or an approved social worker.

    (iii) Two medical recommendations are required:

     (a) A doctor approved under section 12 of the MHA.

     (b) A doctor preferably with previous knowledge of the patient, e.g. the general practitioner.

(2) *Section 4: Admission for assessment in cases of emergency*.

    (i)   This lasts for 72 h.

    (ii)   Application may be made by the nearest relative or preferably by an approved social worker, either of whom must have seen the patient within the previous 24 h.

    (iii) One medical recommendation only is required from a doctor, ideally with prior knowledge of the patient. If this is not possible, it should be clearly stated on the medical recommendation why such a doctor is not available.

ADMINISTRATIVE AND LEGAL CONSIDERATIONS

ACCIDENT AND EMERGENCY RECORDS

The following are guidelines for recording accurate and concise information for every patient examined in the department. Details will obviously vary according to the nature and layout of each department's records. In addition, computerisation of the medical record is being established in many departments, but the same high standards of manual recording must still be adhered to:

(1) Ensure all the boxes at the top of the page have been filled in (usually by the reception staff) to identify the patient fully.

(2) Start by printing your own name, the date and the time you commenced seeing the patient.

(3) Write legibly throughout; other members of staff will be reading your notes which will be meaningless if they are illegible.

(4) Record all the positive clinical findings in the history and examination, and relevant negative findings.

(5) Avoid the use of abbreviations except for unambiguous, approved examples such as BP. Digits should be named not numbered, and Left or Right written in full.

(6) Make detailed notes in assault or traffic accident cases of the patient's recall of events, or from a witness. Document the exact size of bruises or lacerations measured with a ruler.

   (i)   Statements may subsequently be required by the police or a solicitor and could be requested months or even years later, so you cannot rely on your memory!

   (ii)   A photograph is an ideal record and may save a detailed description. Unfortunately few doctors have access to a suitable camera at the necessary time.

(7) Record your diagnosis and differential diagnosis.

(8) Record any investigations performed, and put down the results, including your own interpretation of the x-ray or ECG.

(9) Detail your proposed treatment plan, and carefully record any verbal or written instructions or advice given to the patient.

(10) Record the disposal of the patient:

(i) If you hand the patient over to another A & E department doctor at the end of your shift, record on the notes to whom clinical responsibility has been transferred.

(ii) If you refer to an inpatient team, record the name and seniority of the doctor concerned and the time the patient was referred.

(iii) If the patient is referred to outpatients, record the clinic name and the consultant if possible.

(iv) If the patient is admitted, write the ward and the consultant under whom the patient was admitted on the records.

(v) Finally, if the patient is referred back to the general practitioner, attach a photocopy or carbon copy of any handwritten discharge letter to this doctor onto the A & E record. Computerisation of the medical record may now enable a typed letter to be generated for every patient.

(11) Sign your name clearly at the end of the record, and print your name and initials underneath for future identification.

Most of the above may appear obvious, but it is essential to the quality and continuity of the medical care of the patient. In addition, medicolegal problems are exacerbated by inadequate or incomplete records. Conversely, successful defence of a medical negligence claim may depend on being able to quote from accurate, legible, comprehensive and contemporaneous notes.

COMMUNICATION WITH THE GENERAL PRACTITIONER

It is essential to communicate with the general practitioner by telephone and/or letter as often as possible, particularly in the following circumstances if:

(1) the general practitioner writes a referral letter to you;
(2) you do any tests including bloods, urinalysis, x-ray or ECG, even if they are normal;
(3) you make a new diagnosis;
(4) you start new medication, or change or stop an existing treatment regime;
(5) you refer the patient back to the general practitioner for further care and review, including removing sutures or changing dressings;
(6) you refer the patient to outpatients;
(7) the patient is admitted, or a patient is brought in dead (or dies in the department).

In suitable cases give the patient the letter to deliver by hand, but assume it is likely to be opened and read, so post letters containing sensitive information.

CONSENT

(1) Patients over the age of 16 years may sign or withhold their own informed consent after the doctor has explained the details of the proposed procedure and warned of any possible complications, and the patient understands the implications and nature of the treatment.
(2) In cases of emergency to save life, the doctor should proceed even if consent was not obtained.
(3) Patients under the age of 16 years may be able to consent for treatment provided they have the ability to understand what is proposed, although for major treatment it is preferable to seek consent from the parent or guardian (or teacher in an emergency).
   (i)   If the latter refuse, it is appropriate to request the social work department ask for a magistrate's order to take custody of the child, and thence to grant permission for life-saving treatment such as a blood transfusion in a Jehovah's Witness minor.

SELF-DISCHARGE AND REFUSAL OF TREATMENT

(1) Patients who refuse admission to hospital and a recommended treatment plan should be permitted to discharge themselves after signing the appropriate form, accepting responsibility for their own action.

(2) If they refuse, or disappear before the form is signed, this should be recorded and countersigned by a witness such as a senior nurse or a second doctor.

(3) Patients with conditions which preclude comprehension of the nature and implications of proposed treatment may be given emergency treatment without consent to save life.

(4) Similarly, patients suffering from a mental illness may be detained against their will under the Mental Health Act if they are a danger to themselves or others (see page 372).

POLICE

The police are involved within the A & E department in a number of ways:

(1) *Request for information concerning a patient*:

    (i)   All medical information concerning the care of a patient in the department is confidential and must not be divulged without the patient's written consent.

    (ii)   Traffic police investigating an accident may be told the name, address and age of any patient involved, a brief description of the injury, the severity and disposal, e.g. whether the accident is likely to prove fatal or if the patient is to be admitted or sent home.

    (iii) If a patient is suspected of being involved in a serious arrestable offence such as murder, rape, child abuse or armed robbery, the doctor may disclose this information to a senior police officer, thereby acting in the public interest for the safety of the lives of others.

(iv)   The advice of the senior A & E doctor or hospital administrator should be obtained, if there is any doubt as to the appropriateness of releasing non-clinical information to the police.

(2) *Request to interview a patient*:

(i)   Permission may be granted if the patient is in a fit state medically to be seen, after informing the patient.

(ii)   The doctor may suggest a time limit.

(3) *Request for an alcohol breath test or blood sample*:

(i)   The doctor must first give the police permission to perform these, providing the patient's clinical condition would not be affected detrimentally.

(ii)   In certain circumstances, permission cannot be granted: if the patient is unconscious, critically ill, or incapable of cooperating, possibly due to a facial injury.

(iii)   If permission is granted, inform the patient that you have allowed the police to be involved and record on the A & E record that 'in your opinion the patient was fit to be seen at the time and understood what was happening'.

(iv)   The police officer or police surgeon must take the sample, using all their own equipment, and will not involve the hospital facilities at any stage.

(4) *Request for a police medical statement*:

(i)   The purpose of this statement is to act as a record to be read out in court without requiring the doctor to be present.

(a)   The patient must always provide written consent before you may disclose confidential medical information.

(b)   Use the preprinted forms supplied by the police, which consist of an expenses form, a top sheet and continuation sheets.

(c) State your full name, age, contact address and telephone number, medical qualifications, job status, employing health authority and duration of that employment. State the date you were on duty in the department, the hospital name and the time you examined the patient.

(d) Continue with the full name, age, sex and address of the patient and record the time and date of any subsequent attendances in the A&E department.

(e) The history (as told to you) should be recounted without making personal inferences, and the physical findings recorded, using language a nonmedical person can understand.

(f) The actual size of abrasions, bruises and lacerations should be stated where possible, and a comment made as to whether the injuries found are consistent with the use of a particular weapon or implement as suggested by the patient's history.

(g) List all the investigations performed, including x-rays and laboratory tests and their results.

(h) State the treatment given, including sutures and their number, and record the time the patient spent in hospital or attending outpatients.

(i) Finally, end the report where possible with a prognosis. The report is then signed and countersigned where indicated on each separate page.

(ii) Always keep a photocopy of your report and note the name and number of the police officer requesting the statement, and his police station.

BREAKING THE NEWS OF SUDDEN DEATH

(1) Breaking the news of sudden death to a relative, especially when unexpected as in trauma or cardiac arrest, must be done in the privacy of a quiet relatives room.

(2) Be accompanied by an experienced nurse, introduce yourself, identify the patient's nearest relative and sit by them.

(3) Come to the point avoiding any preamble or euphemisms, and use the words 'dead' or 'death' early on, followed by a brief account of events.

(4) Be prepared to touch or hold the relative's hand and do not be afraid to show concern or empathy yourself. Allow a period of silence, avoiding platitudes or false sympathy but encourage and answer any questions.

(5) Understand that the relative's reaction may vary from numbed silence, disbelief, acute distress to anger, denial and guilt.

(6) Indicate that the nurse can stay with them and when they are ready, encourage them to see and touch the body to say goodbye to their loved one alone.

(7) Ask if the relative wishes the hospital chaplain, social worker or bereavement counsellor contacted. Avoid giving sedative drugs that will only postpone acceptance of what has happened.

(8) Phone the general practitioner and inform the coroner's officer.

(9) Retain the property of the deceased, whatever its condition, for collection by the next-of-kin in accordance with his or her wishes. Avoid then presenting it in a plastic bin bag.

(10) Finally, appreciate the stress and anxiety caused to yourself and the nursing team following an unsuccessful resuscitation. Try to meet together briefly to talk over events and express your own feelings and emotions. Thank everyone for their efforts, particularly the nurse dealing with the relatives and the nurses left to lay out the body.

CORONER

(1) The coroner must be informed of all sudden or unexpected deaths, and deaths involving homicide, suicide, an accident or injury, poisoning, alcohol, surgery, abortion, infancy, neglect, an industrial disease, negligence or patients in police custody.

(2) Thus virtually all patients brought in dead are reported to the coroner; this may be done by the hospital general administration office.

(3) Any patient actually dying in the department should be reported. If there are any suspicious circumstances, this should be done whatever the time of day or night, by contacting the coroner's officer through the local police station (the police are very often involved anyway).

(4) The A & E department doctor is not in a position to sign the death certificate.

ATTENDING AN INQUEST

An inquest takes place in the coroner's court and is purely a fact-finding inquiry, not a trial. It is held in public and the press may be present.

(1) The coroner's officer will inform you of the date, time and place of the inquest. Arrive punctually and suitably dressed. Legal representation may be arranged for you by your medical defence organisation, if on discussion with them they consider it appropriate.

(2) Take the medical notes and a copy of your statement with you. Read both thoroughly beforehand so you have the facts readily available.

(3) The oath is taken, then the coroner will take you through your statement and ask questions.

(4) Your replies should be concise, clear and factual, indicating if they are based on hearsay.

(5) Following this, you may be examined by any 'properly interested persons' or usually their lawyer. You are not obliged to answer any questions that may incriminate you.

(6) After the inquest the coroner's officer will pay you the appropriate witness fee and expenses.

THE MAJOR INCIDENT

(1) Each hospital will have its own plan for coping with large numbers of casualties, known as the Major Disaster Plan.

(2) From this, portions of the plan pertinent to individual members of staff are summarised on documents known as Action Cards. Those concerned with the medical and nursing staff within the department should be distributed to and read by all new members of staff.

(3) All new A & E doctors must also make certain that:

(i)   Switchboard have a reliable contact telephone number for the purpose of an emergency call-out.

(ii)   They know the call-out procedure, the different states of alert and the significance of being the designated hospital or the supporting hospital.

(iii) They understand their role within the department and which senior doctor they are responsible to and from whom they should receive advice.

(iv)   They can operate any equipment reserved for use in a major incident, including that used by the mobile medical team.

(v)   They are familiar with the special stationery and records used in a major incident, including the significance of the triage labels and where to find details of any prehospital care given, particularly drugs and fluids.

(vi)   They know how to obtain social and psychological support following the incident, to minimise the potential for post-traumatic stress.

(4) Some incidents pose an additional danger to staff themselves:

(i) *Radiation contamination*:
- (a) certain hospitals are designated for the care of patients contaminated with radioactive substances;
- (b) however, if a patient requires urgent treatment, they can be taken to the nearest major A & E department;
- (c) advice and help is usually given by a radiation physicist or the local Radiation Protection Advisor;
- (d) staff attending these patients will be assigned to a predetermined isolation and decontamination area, and expected to wear caps, theatre clothes, aprons, double gloves and boots which they should be familiar with in advance.

(ii) *Toxic chemical contamination*:
- (a) the fire brigade are responsible for identifying toxic chemical spillage and decontamination on site usually with large volumes of water;
- (b) similar designated decontamination areas and protective clothing are used by staff as in radiation contamination;
- (c) hypothermia from wet protective blankets must be excluded in all cases, and standard resuscitation procedures adopted without delaying for the arrival of specific antidotes;
- (d) most patients require admission for a period of observation, even if asymptomatic. Inhalation injury and absorption through skin, e.g. of phenol, may cause delayed toxic effects which should be anticipated in advance.

FURTHER READING

Advanced Life Support Group (1993). *Advanced Paediatric Life Support. The Practical Approach*. London: BMJ Publishing Group.

Bacon C. J., Lamb W. H. (1988). *Paediatric Emergencies Diagnosis and Management*, 2nd edn. Oxford: Butterworth-Heinemann.

Bradley J. J. (1986). *The Mental Health Act 1983. The Psychiatric Emergency: Responsibility for Suicidal Patients*. London: The Medical Protection Society Ltd.

Bull P. D. (1991). *Lecture Notes on Diseases of the Ear, Nose and Throat*, 7th edn. Oxford: Blackwell Scientific Publications.

Dreisbach R. H., Robertson W. O. (1987). *Handbook of Poisoning*, 12th edn. Norwalk: Appleton and Lange.

Evans T. R. (1995). *ABC of Resuscitation*, 3rd edn. London: British Medical Journal.

Fulde G. W. O. (1992). *Emergency Medicine: The Principles of Practice*, 2nd edn. Sydney: MacLennan and Petty.

Harwood-Nuss A., Linden C., Luten R., *et al.* (1991). *The Clinical Practice of Emergency Medicine*. Philadelphia: J.B. Lippincott Co.

Harwood-Nuss A., Luten R. (1995). *Handbook of Emergency Medicine*. Philadelphia: J.B. Lippincott Co.

Ho M. T., Saunders C. E. (1990). *Current Emergency Diagnosis and Treatment*, 3rd edn. Norwalk: Appleton and Lange.

Howarth P., Evans R. (1994). *Key Topics in Accident and Emergency Medicine*. Oxford: Bios Scientific Publishers.

Huckstep R. L. (1995). *A Simple Guide to Trauma*, 5th edn. Edinburgh: Churchill Livingstone.

Jenkins J. L., Loscalzo J. L., Braen R. (1995). *Manual of Emergency Medicine*, 3rd edn. Boston: Little, Brown and Co.

Keats T. E. (1989). *Emergency Radiology*, 2nd edn. Chicago: Mosby Year Book Medical Publishers.

Keats T. E. (1991). *Atlas of Normal Roentgen Variants that may Simulate Disease*, 5th edn. Chicago: Mosby Year Book Medical Publishers.

Kilham H. (1993). *The Children's Hospital Handbook*. Camperdown: Sydney. Alken Press Pty. Ltd.

London P. S. (1991). *The Anatomy of Injury and its Surgical Implications*. Oxford: Butterworth-Heinemann.

Mattox K. L. (1994). *Complications of Trauma*. New York: Churchill Livingstone.

McLatchie G. R. (1993). *Essentials of Sports Medicine*, 2nd edn. Edinburgh: Churchill Livingstone.

McRae R. (1994). *Practical Fracture Treatment*, 3rd edn. Edinburgh: Churchill Livingstone.

Mengert T., Eisenberg M. S., Copass M. K. (1995). *Emergency Medical Therapy*, 4th edn. Philadelphia: W. B. Saunders.

Mirvis S. E., Young J. W. R. (1992). *Imaging in Trauma and Critical Care*. Baltimore: Williams and Wilkins.

Oh T. E. (1990). *Intensive Care Manual*, 3rd edn. Sydney: Butterworth-Heinemann.

Proudfoot A. T. (1993). *Acute Poisoning Diagnosis and Management*, 2nd edn. Oxford: Butterworth-Heinemann.

Raby N., Berman L., de Lacy G. (1995). *Accident and Emergency Radiology*. Philadelphia: W. B. Saunders Co.

Richards A. B. *Ocular Emergencies*. Romford: Smith & Nephew Pharmaceuticals Ltd.

Roberts J. R., Hedges J. R. (1991). *Clinical Procedures in Emergency Medicine*, 2nd edn. Philadelphia: W.B. Saunders Co.

Robertson C., Redmond A. D. (1994). *The Management of Major Trauma*, 2nd edn. Oxford: Oxford University Press.

Robinson R., Stott R. (1993). *Medical Emergencies Diagnosis and Management*, 6th edn. Oxford: Butterworth-Heinemann.

Rosen P., Barkin R., *et al.* (1992). *Emergency Medicine. Concepts and Clinical Practice*, 3rd edn. St Louis: Mosby Year Book.

Rubenstein D., Wayne D. (1991). *Lecture Notes on Clinical Medicine*, 4th edn. Oxford: Blackwell Scientific Publications.

Rutherford W. H., Illingworth R. N., Marsden A. K., *et al.* (1989). *Accident and Emergency Medicine*, 2nd edn. Edinburgh: Churchill Livingstone.

Settle J. A. D. (1987). *Burns – The First Five Days*. Romford: Smith and Nephew Pharmaceuticals Ltd.

Skinner D., Driscoll P., Earlham R. (1991). *ABC of Major Trauma*. London: British Medical Journal.

Sprigings D., Chambers J. (1995). *Acute Medicine: A Practical Guide to the Management of Medical Emergencies*, 2nd edn. Oxford: Blackwell Scientific Publications.

Steedman D. J. (1994). *Environmental Medical Emergencies*. Oxford: Oxford University Press.

The Medical Defence Union (1991). *A & E Risk Management*. London: The Medical Defence Union.

The Medical Defence Union (1993). *Issues in Medical Defence. Medico-Legal Issues in Clinical Practice*, 2nd edn. London: The Medical Defence Union Ltd.

The Medical Defence Union (1992). *Medical Records*. London: The

Medical Defence Union Ltd.

Tinker J., Jones S. N. (1990). *A Pocket Book for Intensive Care*, 2nd edn. London: Edward Arnold.

Tintinalli J., Krome R., Ruiz E. (1992). *Emergency Medicine. A Comprehensive Study Guide*, 3rd edn. New York: McGraw-Hill.

Trevor-Roper P. D. (1986). *Lecture Notes on Ophthalmology*, 7th edn. Oxford: Blackwell Scientific Publications.

Trunkey D. D., Lewis F. R. (1991). *Current Therapy of Trauma*, 3rd edn. Toronto: B. C. Decker Inc.

Webb L. A. (1995). *Eye Emergencies Diagnosis and Management*. Oxford: Butterworth-Heinemann.

Westaby S. (1985). *Wound Care*. Oxford: Butterworth-Heinemann.

Westaby S. (1989). *Trauma: Pathogenesis and Treatment*. Oxford: Butterworth-Heinemann.

Willatts S. M., Winter R. J. (1992). *Principles and Protocols in Intensive Care*. London: Farrand Press.

GLOSSARY

A&E	accident and emergency
AC	alternating current
ACE	angiotensin-converting enzyme
ACTH	adrenocorticotrophic hormone
AIDS	acquired immune deficiency syndrome
ANF	antinuclear factor
AP	anteroposterior
ATLS	Advanced Trauma Life Support
b.d.	*bis in die* (Latin: twice daily)
BIPP	bismuth and iodoform paraffin paste
BNF	British National Formulary
BP	blood pressure
°C	degrees Celsius
C1:C7	first and seventh cervical vertebrae
C7:T1	seventh cervical and first thoracic vertebrae
CCU	coronary care unit
CD4+	cluster designation (of antigen) 4+
CDC	Centers for Disease Control and Prevention
CK	creatine phosphokinase
CK-MB	creatine phosphokinase MB isoenzymes
Cl	chloride
cm	centimetre
CNS	central nervous system
CO_2	carbon dioxide
CPR	cardiopulmonary resuscitation
CSF	cerebrospinal fluid
CT	computerised (axial) tomography
CVA	cerebrovascular accident
CVP	central venous pressure
CXR	chest x-ray
D&C	dilatation and curettage
DC	direct current
DKA	diabetic ketoacidosis
DNA	deoxyribonucleic acid
DoH	Department of Health
DPL	diagnostic peritoneal lavage
DVT	deep vein thrombosis
ECG	electrocardiogram
e.g.	*exempli gratia* (Latin: for example)

EMD	electromechanical dissociation
ENT	ear, nose and throat
ERPC	evacuation of retained products of conception
ESR	erythrocyte sedimentation rate
ET	endotracheal
etc.	*et cetera* (Latin: and the rest)
°F	degrees Fahrenheit
FBC	full blood count
g	gram
G&S	group and save (blood)
GCS	Glasgow Coma Scale
g/dl	grams per decilitre
GI	gastrointestinal
Glucostix	enzyme-impregnated reagent strips for measuring capillary blood glucose
GP	general practitioner
GTN	glyceryl trinitrate
h	hour
H_1/H_2	histamine type 1/histamine type 2
Hb	haemoglobin
HCG	human chorionic gonadotrophin
HCO_3	bicarbonate
HIV	human immunodeficiency virus
HLA	human leucocyte antigen
HMSO	Her Majesty's Stationery Office
HTIG	human tetanus immunoglobulin
ICS	intercostal space
i.e.	*id est* (Latin: that is)
IgE	immunoglobulin E
i.m.	intramuscular
ITU	intensive therapy unit
IUCD	intrauterine contraceptive device
i.v.	intravenous
IVU	intravenous urogram
J	joule
JVP	jugular venous pressure
K	potassium
KCl	potassium chloride
kg	kilogram
KUB	kidneys, ureters, bladder
l	litre
LBBB	left bundle branch block
LFTs	liver function tests
l/min	litres per minute

LP	lumbar puncture
LSD	lysergic acid diethylamide
MAST	military antishock trousers
mEq/l	milliequivalents per litre
mg	milligram
μg	microgram
MHA	Mental Health Act
min	minute
MI	myocardial infarction
ml	millilitre
mm	millimetre
mmHg	millimetres of mercury
mmol	millimole
mmol/l	millimoles per litre
MCP	metacarpophalangeal
MSU	midstream specimen of urine
Mu	megaunit
Na	sodium
NAI	nonaccidental injury
NG	nasogastric
ng	nanogram
normal saline	isotonic 0.9% sodium chloride solution
NSAID	nonsteroidal anti-inflammatory drug
OM	occipitomental
OPG	orthopantomogram
PA	postero-anterior
$PaCO_2$	partial pressure of carbon dioxide (arterial)
PCV	packed cell volume
PE	pulmonary embolus
PEF	peak expiratory flow
PGL	persistent generalised lymphadenopathy
pH	negative logarithm of the hydrogen ion concentration
PaO_2	partial pressure of oxygen (arterial)
PPF	plasma protein fraction
PTA	post-traumatic amnesia
PTI	prothrombin index
p.r.	per rectum
q.d.s.	*quater in die sumendus* (Latin: four times daily)
RBBB	right bundle branch block
rt-PA	recombinant tissue plasminogen activator
s	seconds
s.c.	subcutaneous
SCIWORA	spinal cord injury without radiological abnormality

SCUBA	self-contained underwater breathing apparatus
SLR	straight-leg raising
TB	tuberculosis
t.d.s	*ter in die sumendus* (Latin: three times daily)
TIA	transient ischaemic attack
U	unit
U&E	urea and electrolytes
UK	United Kingdom
USA	United States of America
UTI	urinary tract infection
VF	ventricular fibrillation
VT	ventricular tachycardia
WCC	white cell count
X-match	cross-match blood

Index